# LIVING BETTER WITH HYPOTHYROIDISM

A PATIENTS EXPERIENCE

STEP BY STEP SELF HELP GUIDELINES

## HOW **YOU** CAN MANAGE YOUR ILLNESS AND FEEL WELLNESS

BY

# SUSAN SEYMOUR

*Incorporating "Living with Hypothyroidism" Books One and Two First published 1999*

# DISCLAIMER

Neither the publisher, nor the author, nor any health practitioner quoted in this book take any consequences from any procedure, treatment, dietary modifications, action or application of medication or preparation by any person reading or following the information in this book. The publication of this book does not in any way constitute the practice of medicine, and the book does not in any way attempt to replace the advice and treatment of your doctor, physician or pharmacist. Before undertaking any treatment the author and publisher advise you to consult your doctor, or health practitioner regarding any prescription or treatment and therapies that may be beneficial for your particular health problems, and the dosages that may be best for you. Neither the author nor publisher takes any responsibility for your health on an individual basis. The contents of the book are designed to advise generally. What suits one person will not suit another; we are all individuals.

Printed and bound in the U. K. and on e-books
London
First published January, 1999
Revised and re-printed 2nd edition October 2000
Revised and re-printed 3rd edition, February 2001
Re-printed 2002
Revised and re-issued 2014

## Author's Note

A self help book for those suffering from
hypothyroidism with guidelines on self healing

My personal experiences, research and training
from 1996 to date in hormones, diet, lifestyle and
emotional stress.

How you can manage the illness of hypothyroidism

Each person is different and should be treated as
an individual.

# CONTENTS – Part One

# <u>CONTENTS</u> – Part Two

# ALPHABETICAL INDEX OF TERMS AND EXPLANATIONS

# INTRODUCTION

Living with hypothyroidism is something that 99% of hypothyroids do. The purpose of this book is to enable the reader to understand that it is possible to live a better standard of life. More importantly that you can become euthyroid - which is neither hypo (under-active), nor hyper (overactive) by making some changes to your everyday living.

The intentions of this book are to give an overview of the hypothyroid illness, it may, as you read on, put you into this classification, or it may not. The information included is available in more detail from the reading list. The hope of the author is that the contents of this book encourages you to go forward and research what you believe may be your illness.

Would you like to have a stable weight? Be a happy outgoing individual? Have energy and vitality? Be emotionally balanced? Let us hope the following pages are an introduction to understanding what happens to you when you are hypothyroid and why. More importantly how you can change your life by taking control of it. No one can heal you except you.

My problems began with a car accident. This was followed by two major surgical operations. Sadly the next trauma came the following year with the death of my beloved grandparents. Finally I fell ill with meningitis. Any one of these could have triggered hypothyroidism. An excess of pharmaceutical HRT put the final touches to my illness. I've been prescribed anti-depressants, sleeping tablets, antibiotics, blood tests and had more visits to the doctor during the early nineties than in the rest of my life put together. The symptoms listed later in the information pack pretty much totally described me. I felt despair.

In 1996 I was sitting in a slimming clinic, (no the tablets did not work!), when I read an article in She magazine. I read of hypothyroid symptoms, which described me to a T. At the end there was a help line number. I wrote it down ... and, as you do when you are not ready for something, it sat in my purse for months. Like many other hypothyroids I placed my trust in the NHS and persisted steadfastly through the system to the top. I was told many things but the final straw came when our local head of endocrinology told me that my weight gain was from (1) eating too much - I was in my fifth month of an 800 calorie diet, (2) I should exercise more - I did 30 minutes of aerobics each morning five days a week, and (3) It was in my genes - I told him that none of my family were excessively overweight, quite the opposite. Finally to cap matters I was most certainly NOT hypothyroid as my blood tests said so! They were borderline; (10). No one ever explained to me the risks of taking pharmaceutical HRT, the effects it would have on my liver and insulin levels, or the risk of death from thrombosis. More importantly I was not told it would downgrade my thyroid. Why I was not told I wondered? I realize now that doctors get no special training in thyroid problems. If I had been CLINICALLY diagnosed and treated correctly my life would have been transformed. You cannot treat a blood test.

During the last seventeen years I have read many books; researched constantly, discussed the thyroid problem with doctors, and many thousand patients. I have listened carefully and come to the following conclusion. <u>People will act on their illness when they</u> <u>are ready</u>. You may, like I was initially, be swayed by various non-believers. You may not want to try the advice. (Many people actually do like being ill - believe it or not). Many are told of out of date practices and until they, (as one lady said recently); "Hit that brick wall". And they will continue to be ill. It is up to the individual. As you are reading this book you are a step closer to helping yourself. You cannot rely solely on others to make you well. Your others may just like your dependency on them and try to keep you ill to feed their own needs.

My brick wall was the coughing up of blood, half a cup at first. "How long have you had the cough?" the doctor locum asked. Through the blood soaked hankie I croaked that I did not have a cough, and that I was coughing because of the blood. I could see in his eyes he did not believe me, and by his body language – he was slouched on my sofa – and that he was unconvinced. A chest X-ray followed the following week - it was O.K. I had no infection. Things got much worse. I couldn't sleep lying flat - well if the truth be told I couldn't get to sleep at all. I lay down exhausted each night, and almost at once my heart began to race, nothing eased the lack of falling into deep REM sleep. Believe me I tried everything from Nytol to conventional sleeping tablets. They made me feel worse. The lump in my throat felt like a large marble. The inability to swallow properly made me fear I was soon to be dead. I was miserable, unhappy, getting bigger, exhausted and afraid. This was my brick wall.

It was August, some six months later that I finally called the number in my purse. A sweet lady called Caroline talked to me for about an hour. She suggested another number for me to call to check my symptoms. I called Diana, another understanding lady, "Yes", she said I had most of the symptoms and finally "Did I want to see the doctor?" My grateful reply was of course "Yes please". I thought 'At last someone who knows what they are doing'. The following week I drove to Leeds and along with lots of other people attended the private clinic.

So then what happened you might ask? After a long wait (they had kindly squeezed my appointment in), my turn came around eventually.

Firstly my details were taken, and a glass thermometer was popped under my armpit. My thyroid - for the first time - was gently fingertip examined. I knew that by now it was the size of a small golf ball - swollen and hard. The doctor made a note of my under arm temperature, my pulse, and then checked my blood pressure, (although I do not recall him doing the sitting standing blood pressure test for the adrenals). He looked intently at my swollen tongue, my moon shaped swollen face, and at my puffy sore eyes. "Yes he said I had a thyroid problem – and he was right". He told me to stop taking HRT, as "the menopause was not an illness", (I was so young and had no ovaries by this time). Then he prescribed 25mgs of Thyroxine for me ......... and at first I felt really hellish. My body closed down and went into repair and recovery state. On the low doses I could not function, and was in fact worse. It went on for too long, what should have taken a week took another month. My thyroid stimulating hormone, (TSH), had almost shut down, and my pituitary had stopped making the stimulating hormone because of the induced welfare state by Thyroxine. I had to wait for another month on this low dose, why I will never know as it is dangerous to be on low doses, and did not begin to feel better until it increased.

However things were still not right. I tried to go for a walk one-day -something I had no problem with as a rule, as I have been into fitness all my life. I was so exhausted I could hardly move, never mind walk. Upon my return home I telephoned the doctor in a panic. At no time were my adrenals discussed. I also told him about the burning feeling in my brain. He was unaware of this and seemed bewildered. I now realize when the adrenals decline the thyroid usually falls soon after. If you treat the thyroid and not the adrenals exhaustion can be the result.

At another visit to the private clinic I was prescribed Armour, pork thyroid, which after Thyroxine (Synthroid), I thought was wonderful. (I now know only 6 people in 100 who test well for Thyroxine, and Armour can also be toxic to some people). One again the dose was low, however because it contains all the thyroid hormones it was a huge improvement. My pulse slowly began to rise, from 35C, but my hair started falling out, and the energy levels were still poor.

People commented that I looked like I had lost weight because my face lost its' moon shape. The puffiness has almost gone. It was six months before my brain even began to come out of the oxygen starved fog, however on Thyroxine I became slightly dyslexic. For those who wrote to me after the media publications some would see an added letter occasionally. Aand was my favourite for some reason my brain happily added an extra 'A' when it should not have.

Recovery was slow - it takes six months to even

start to feel better. Usually the cells take two years to heal, even longer for your liver, which is the last to heal.

I had various strange changes to my body, some are listed above. One of the most important to me was my tummy measured ten inches less than it had before the thyroid treatment. Needless to say I was happy that it no longer resembled Buddha. My bottom was five inches less. My waist three inches less. Overall from ten points of my body I had lost thirty inches. However my body did some frightening things, for example I had red eyes for three months, (low adrenals), they were so bad that my optician was concerned and carefully tested them. My saliva glands changed, my mouth was very dry, sometimes having an odd metallic taste. I remember that my nails and hair were the first to change. My hair had bounce again and was no longer lank, it had a new shine. Strong nails grew which were pink and not pale. The hard skin on my feet was gone by month four. I noticed I could sing again by month six. The frightening lump had almost gone in my throat. It was when I changed to natural thyroid that I really began to get better.

Life has moved on a few years since that time. I visited a new private doctor who told me that I have a T4 to T3 conversion problem. He prescribed T3 - Tertroxin twice a day. (Read more about conversion later.) I now felt that I could cope with going out. Other significant improvements were also made for example I no longer feel frightened by night driving. (The two black dots that were before my eyes instead of the road have long gone). However regulation of my hormones was haphazard to say the least. This was possibly due to the length of my thyroid starvation, or more probably the lack of ovaries. I am unsure if I will ever regain my full health, but life is much better. I still have to pace myself, and have painfully learnt the art of health management, learning what suits me and what works for me.

The inception of the support group in 1998 has taught me many lessons. One of the most important is that far too many people, (like me), place their trust in their doctors and not enough in themselves. Since the 1950's, when blood tests came into full use, the tried and tested methods of evaluating hypothyroidism have been largely ignored. A blood test is only a snapshot in time and in most cases will not be 100% accurate. It certainly will not make you well. A blood test cannot accurately describe what is going on in your body, it cannot differentiate between primary, secondary and third-rate hypothyroidism. It cannot evaluate the interaction between your total hormone balance and only 9%, yes that is nine, have been proved to be accurately diagnosed in this illness. In fact, at the time of writing, the last survey undertaken by the Audit Commission into laboratories shows that only 50% of them in this country supply accurate results. That is half!

So what happens next?  How do you go about finding out (one) is it your thyroid or (two) your adrenals dropping causing your thyroid problems? Is it the medication you are taking? For example it could be anti-depressants.  Is it foods that are affecting you? (They are usually half the cause; and half the healing). Do you have emotional problems? These could be grief, divorce or anything.  The following is a simple to follow course of suggestion on how you may discover you current health state. Then how do you go about solving the problem of your illness?  What steps can you take to help yourself?  Do you even want to be well?  The answers may be found in the following chapters. These are not meant to replace conventional medicine, but to supplement it in a way that you can understand.

## **<u>THE MORNING</u>**

Buy a thermometer from a chemist, pharmacy or drugstore; they do not cost much, and are vital for monitoring your health.  The night before shake it down.  If you have old mercury one, do take care not to smash it on the bedside table.  Upon waking in bed, while you are still warm and relaxed, and before getting up, tuck the thermometer under your armpit snugly; place the bulb nearest to skin.  Wait for ten minutes. It does take that amount of time for the tissue test.  Write the result down in a notebook.  Most thermometers are marked either in red or with a mark at the normal level - which is 98.4F or 37 centigrade. If you have a consecutively low temperature below 97.8F or 36.6C, you appear to be hypothyroid – or you could be hypo-adrenal. This test is called The Barnes Temperature Test and is used worldwide for metabolic disorders. (Dr. Broda Barnes was one of the worlds leading thyroid experts).

The Three Checks – step one

When you have been up for an hour, and been pottering about, take your pulse for a whole minute. You do this be placing two fingers flat to the inside of your wrist. Do not use your thumb as it has its' own pulse. The resting pulse is usually around 70 beats per minute. The pottering around pulse is usually 80 – 84 beats per minute. Write it down next to the date and your temperature. Later in the day take it again. An aerobic pulse should be over 90 beats per minute; if you are hyperthyroid it will usually be over 91 beats per minute. Most hypothyroids have a pulse of 65 or less. Many have such a weak pulse they cannot measure it. Try your neck instead of your wrist if this happens. Follow the jaw down from the ear until you feel the pulse. Don't forget to write it down next to your temperature along with the date and time. If your pulse is 20 beats below then you are probably getting that percentage less of oxygen to the tissues. A low pulse is the body's way of saving energy it does not have, a survival mode.

## Step Two

Weigh yourself, again write it down. There is a good reason for this. You may have food allergies; this causes the tissues to bloat with fluid, hence increased weight. Wheat, grains, seeds, carbohydrates, yeasts and sugars are the main culprits, (see "A Thyroid and Hormone Diet").

## Step Three

If you have a weight problem it is a good idea to measure ten points of your body beginning with your neck and working down.

It is <u>very important to have breakfast</u>. I know you may have no appetite, but you must remember food is fuel - which is heat and energy. My starvation diet did me no good at all; it increased my weight by 4 stones in as many months. Don't go for artificial stimulants like coffee and tea. Do not eat exhausting and acid foods like grains and sugar. Sugar poisoning is explained in the book "Primitive Healing". You need protein and oils. Bacon and eggs with any good oil, or two fried eggs in butter or grape seed oil

If you are on thyroid therapy take your medication now with boiled spring water. If it sends you to sleep take at night. T3 should not be taken at night the energy hormone keeps you awake.

If you are on thyroid homeopathic take it upon waking and before breakfast, after doing the three checks/tests. Remember homeopathic medicine is very powerful, and it acts slowly and gently on cell memory.

The next part may suprise you. If you are extremely exhausted the brain may be short of glucose. You can begin with a glass of freshly squeezed organic apple juice mixed with half a teaspoonful of glucose. You can dilute this half and half with boiled spring water. (Glucose is NOT sugar, it is the fuel your brain and cells live on and hypothyroids usually have a glucogenisis problem- i.e. they cannot convert food into glucose). Many have low blood sugar because the thyroid stimulates the pancreas and the digestive system. Hypoglycemia is common in this illness. Do NOT use orange or grapefruit as they can interfere with other medication and some blood groups are toxic to them. Remember that citrus fruit is digested further down in the gut, and needs to have ten minutes for digestion before adding more food into the gut. Grapefruit is a stimulant. Grapefruit juice and glucose is a good pick me up and many group members feel better for taking it three times a day. If you are blood group O do not take grapefruit or orange in any form **any time**. Finish off with a cup of herb tea, or thyroid tea, one to suit you from the list at the end of this book. Make this with boiled mineral water. A word of caution – make sure the

18

mineral water has low nitrates and NO fluoride added.

It is important to eat regularly if you are hypothyroid. You will NOT loose weight unless you do because your metabolism needs food to function. Have something small that would cover the palm of your hand every two hours, (not wheat, grains or sugars).

Breakfast may be late in the morning because many hypothyroids sleep poorly, (I did not see eleven o' clock a.m. for many years). However this changes with correct medication. If you wake up and do not have energy then it could be a liver problem. Increasing oils usually helps this – the liver is stimulated by proteins, fats and oils. T4 to T3 cannot properly occur without oils as the conversion takes place mostly in the liver.

Two hours later, have something small like natural yoghurt, nuts or berries. You need protein and some fat because all hormones are made from cholesterol.

Before the morning snack if you are able, do a little yoga. If you are a newly recovering patient take it slowly. The breathing exercises are especially excellent. Take your time; begin at five minutes and build up monthly as you begin to heal. Remember if you have breakfast at nine to do this and hour before you have your eleven o' clock snack.  Yoga videos have specialist exercises for thyroid.

At midday go for a fiften minute walk to maximise vitamin D from the sun.

## THE AFTERNOON

Unless you have grade one, (very serious) hypothyroidism you will probably be pottering about at home or working if you can.  For those of you who have low adrenals you may be confined to the sofa.

Lunch should contain one third protein, oils, at least an ounce, and vegetables or salad.

At some point in the afternoon try and walk for twenty minutes in a green place - preferably not near traffic - but in a low pollution area.  The beach is excellent because the crashing waves release minerals and energy, which is beneficial for us.

A mid afternoon snack can alternate with a morning snack.

If you feel tired then go to sleep.  When you sleep you make hormones. One of these is growth hormone, (a liver stimulant), in early stages of sleep.  G.H. (growth hormone) interacts with the thyroid and makes it work properly.  This is one of the reasons you may feel tired all the time if your thyroid is too low. Carbohydrates exhaust this pathway. In order for the hypothalamus-gallbladder pathway to flow you need to get enough rest. One of the mistakes hypothyroids make is not allowing the healing cycle to take place. Instead of resting, and allowing the healing to take place at its' own pace, people often fight against it. The body needs balance and rest to heal. Avoid stimulants like caffeine, alcohol, drugs and smoking or heavy exercise.

## **TEA TIME**

Make a meal, which is one third meat or fish and two thirds low carb vegetables, and drink herb teas or boiled spring water. The food should cover the size of your open hand, one third protein, the size of your palm and two thirds vegetables the size of your fist. If the rest of the family is NOT hypothyroid add small amounts of carbohydrates for them. Take care to avoid cruciferous vegetables, which inhibit thyroid function.

**\*\*IMPORTANT NOTE** – THESE ARE SIMPLE GUIDELINES – HOWEVER NOT ALL FOODS SUIT ALL PEOPLE, AND YOU SHOULD BE TESTED BEFORE EMBARKING ON THIS REGIME. Blood group 'O' are most affected by modern foods and are the most likely to develop hypothyroidism.

# NIGHT TIME

If you are not lactose, (milk sugar) intolerant, or have a dairy allergy do drink a glass of warm milk and/or lettuce before bedtime. Milk raises calcium levels and helps sleep. Lettuce is a natural sedative. Coral calcium helps balance the pH of the body. It is said that it helps to lose weight too. If you take thyroid supplements you should take calcium, it is the most deficient of all the supplements. High strength amino acids also can help you to sleep, in particular L-Ornithine. Many on a high grain diet are amino acid deficient.

It is common for hypothyroids to be exhausted as they get into bed. As soon as their heads hit the pillow it becomes another story, as I can testify. The heart rate picks up, even palpitations start. The brain will not go to sleep, because stage 4 deep REM sleep eludes those with this illness. You may become nocturnal. I remember many mornings finally getting off to sleep at eight a.m. Many nights sat watching television. Sleeping pills cause a dull mental state, which must be how senility feels. If the liver is not functioning correctly they will be just another toxin to add to an already stressed body. Another hormone, cortisol, is also important for a good nights sleep.

Warmth is essential. While you are awake you can regulate your body temperature by adding, and

22

shedding clothing.  If you have first or secondary hypothyroidism you may also have a failing or struggling pituitary gland.  This gland in your brain sends messages for hormone regulation, and through negative feedback is controlled by the hypothalamus.  The hypothalamus also regulates temperature.  You can tell if this gland is working properly by taking your temperature, most hypothyroids have low levels.  Don't be afraid to wrap up at night in thermals, or perhaps wear two or three loose thin layers to keep your body heat in.  Be careful not to get your neck chilled – always wear a silk scarf in the cold.  Have a low pillow so that the blood is not restricted to the neck by bending it too much.  Do not have electricity near to your head.  Have your bed with the head facing north if you live in the northern hemisphere.

If you wake up through the night have milk or calcium to help you get back to sleep.  Calcium is vital, I cannot stress this enough.  More about how this is critical in the book Primitive Healing.  You may also have an adrenal and/or natural progesterone problem.  Men need help with these too.  Snoring is another prime indicator of low thyroid, to the point of breath holding for long periods of time.

Alcohol and smoking make having a good nights sleep worse.

# HORMONES

Some of your most common questions and my
answers

Are you taking pharmaceutical HRT?  Do you know
what it does?  Do you know how it affects the other
parts of your body?  Why do 78% of women give it
up within six months, and the other twenty percent
within six years?  Why does it make us fat?  Do I
agree that in theory is one of the 20th century
breakthroughs – the answer is yes.  Do I feel the
pharmaceutical companies have the combination
balance wrong?  The answer is usually yes I do.
How it is delivered to the patient gives me great
cause for concern.  Would I say that we have got it
totally wrong in the U.K.? – answer everyone is
different.  Could it be better – answer yes, much
better.  Do men feel the same way about
testosterone?  Answer no.  Why?  It stimulates the
thyroid where oestrogen overloads and downgrades
it.  Do the physicians get the females hormone
meds right? – answer no.  Why? They are of the
opinion that natural progesterone is only needed if
you are ovulating or have a womb.  Where does
natural progesterone come from if you do not have
any ovaries?  Answer the adrenals.  Remember men
make oestrogen and progesterone too. Women have
around 10% of testosterone.

I really feel more research should be done as our
hormones are messengers of the body, telling it

how to work properly.

This takes us on to the endocrine system and its' functions:

PITUITARY GLAND

In the brain at the top of our spines is a bone, which holds the pituitary gland.  The pituitary itself is about the size of a pea.  It is connected to the hypothalmus by a stalk.  The two interact between each other and act as a regulating mechanism for senses and functions of the body.

The pituitary has two sections - the anterior pituitary and the posterior pituitary.

The anterior pituitary makes growth hormone, thyroid stimulating hormone (TSH), Adrenocorticotrophic hormone, follicle-stimulating hormone (FSH), lutenizing hormone (LH), prolactin, and melanogyte hormone (MSH)

The posterior pituitary makes antidiuretic hormone (ADH) and Oxytocin.

A simplified explanation of these:

**_Growth hormone_** controls body size, carbohydrate metabolism, skin function, liver function, conversion of T4 to T3 and it interacts with the thyroid to stimulate it work properly.  One if its' key functions is to control glucogenesis. It is a master player and is totally ignored by the medical profession. Carbohydrates and starches exhaust and drain our levels of GH.

**_TSH, thyroid stimulating hormone_** controls thyroid output, including the parathyroids, which regulate calcium conversion to bone. **_ACTH_** stimulates adrenal function. **_FSH_** in women development of ovarian follicle and secretion of oestrogen, in men sperm production LH induces ovulation and stimulates natural progesterone production, in men stimulates androgen production in adrenals.

**_Prolactin_** produces milk in breasts MSH_darkens and colour of our skin ADH affects water absorption and the kidneys Oxytocin_contracts uterus and stimulates the flow of milk.

What can go wrong with the pituitary? It can become swollen or it can shrink, this is called atrophy. Aspartame in cordials, yogurt, fizzy drinks, and processed foods cause pituitary problems and brain tumours. Pregnancy causes the pituitary to swell. After giving birth in some women it does not go down. Checks should be made on: pulse rate, blood pressure, is the skin dehydrated? (Try the pinch test, if the skin on the back of the hand when pinched goes down too slowly you may be dehydrated). Is the skin elastic or oily? How about your body hair distribution?

Look carefully at your nails – is there thickness, brittleness, and softness?  Do your breasts feel tender, are you lactating?   Your voice is also a good indicator and patient's speech should be listened to for huskiness, slurring of words, poor memory upon recall, hoarseness of voice and pitch. You may be unable to sing where you had no problems before.

Chemicals also damage this delicate gland, condtioner, perfumes etc. all affect it.  Hair dye can be a major caus of hypothyroidism and hypo-pituitaryism.  Try to be as naural as possible.

HYPOTHALAMUS

All of the pituitary hormones have releasing hormones in the hypothalamus - **_GnRH_** releases FSH and LH.  **_GHRH_** releases growth hormone. **_SS_** inhibits GH and TSH. **_TRH_** releases TSH and prolactin. **_PIH_** inhibits prolactin. **_PRH_** releases prolactin. **_CRH_** releases ACTH to secrete cortisol.

The balance of the body is regulated by these releasing and inhibiting hormones.  If one goes wrong it has a knock on effect throughout the endocrine system.

The hypothalamus controls the endocrine system using negative feedback.  When a hormone is too high it makes the reverse hormone to stop the production.  This is why often doctors only check

TSH, thyroid stimulating hormone as a measure of thyroid function. Of course it has little to do with cellular function or metabolism.

THYROID

The thyroid is a butterfly shaped gland sitting astride the trachea below and next to the larynx /voice box. The thyroid hormones are formed by the amino acid L-tyrosine, (Aspartame interferes with this), and iodine. There are two hormones T4 which has four 'ears' of iodine and T3 which has three. T3 is up to five times more concentrated that T4. There is also a protein compound called thyroglobulin. If you have no ovaries then you may have a conversion problem because of this. The thyroid oxygenates the cells of the body. It helps them to reproduce healthily and evenly. Thyroxine is only part of the output of the gland, and for normal function natural thyroid, (dried) is much better. It was used extremely well for almost a century before Glaxo introduced Thyroxine. They did a sterling marketing job of getting the doctors to prescribe it instead of natural thyroid. Saying it was better because it was purer. So much so that in the mid 1980's the NIMS took it out of the directory. (More on thyroid history, and development in part two of this book; formerly "Living with Hypothyroidism Book Two"). If a product is not listed in the current NIMS then doctors will not usually prescribe it. Natural thyroid has all the hormones and proteins where

Thyroxine does not. Thyroxine reduces TSH to virtually nil, (usually in the TSH test to 0.03), where natural does not. Natural works in harmony with the hypothalamus and Thyroxine may not.

Doctors work on the theory that in primary hypothyroidism if TSH is elevated then there is a problem, and vice versa. They do not have many (or any), theories for secondary or third-rate hypothyroidism. Many doctors ONLY test for TSH, to see if the thyroid is struggling.

Often incorrect blood tests are done - they should be FT4, TSH and FT3 - F being free i.e. the amount of free T4/T3 in the bloodstream, unbound by proteins or oestrogen. Another complication is that the labs often use different testing methods, systems and ranges throughout the country and the world. It is no wonder everyone is confused. From the feedback I receive a large majority of patients are told that they are 'normal' or 'borderline'. Few are diagnosed clinically, (upon symptoms). Even less have a gentle fingertip examination. When patients first ask for their test results the answer is almost universal - normal. No one ever asks for a copy of their results without being prompted. In any case too many other hormones interfere with the tests for them to be reliable. In some cases the borderline and normal results are accurate as the adrenals are causing the problem. The adrenals can drop first and the thyroid follows afterwards. It is quite common for the patient to be treated incorrectly in my and many others opinions, by waiting for the thyroid to drop below the baseline then treating it without supporting the adrenals. This is something thyroid specialists have been explaining to the medical profession for years. Their challenge to conventional protocols sadly forced them into retirement as an alternative to being struck off. The bottom line is that a blood test will not make you well. It is morally wrong for a doctor to treat a blood test and not a person. The move towards the current requirements of "evidence based" medicine, (a quote from Dr. Toft of the British Thyroid Foundation), is haphazard to say the least, and it is generally due to cost that the true cause of this illness is never discovered.

## **An explanation about medication**

Guidelines given by world experts are that the **BASIC** level for an adult human being is 125mcgs of Thyroxine. The average dose is 150mcgs. However no one takes weight into consideration. Initially this works if administered in a sensible way. The dose should begin at 50mcgs and be increased on a 25mcgs bi-weekly basis UNTIL THE PATIENT FEELS WELL AND IS SLIGHTLY under HYPERTHYROID, (called euthyroid neither over nor under). This is rarely done. Many people try to control their own medication, (self dosing), by taking their temperature each morning and pulse at lunchtime. The part of the equation they miss is that on average Thyroxine _takes three - four days to get into the cells and three - four days to get out_. So if you are like the former National Health lady Nona you should know that if you overdose, as she did, you will probably finish up in hospital, she told me she took over 200mcgs of Thyroxine one day, (I will not say the actual correct amount), which is downright dangerous, and could have had dire consequences. Was this a cry for help, desperation or in her case, as someone who should have known better, or just stupid?

It is only when you reach the normal temperature and pulse that you should begin to heal and get well. It is usually around six months before you begin to improve in a significant way, although some people do improve quickly by getting their foods right. Still this does not happen overnight. On the contrary it takes at least two years for all your cells to heal, along with your immune system, your nerves, and lastly your organs.

Taking thyroid medication is not like taking an Asprin - you don't feel well an hour later. Incidentally Asprin stops the thyroid from working by inhibiting the binding process. Long term Thyroxine often hits problems. Because TSH is reduced to almost nil a conversion problem happens. The liver begins to struggle because of the inhibition of stimulating hormone, (the thyroid not needing it) and also growth hormone is inhibited. When GH is too low so is liver function.

Poor liver function equals poor T3 conversion. T3 is the energy hormone. Some people do better on T3 only.

I know both from personal experience and feedback from people that low levels of Thyroxine make one feel hellish. My calcium conversion was low and my nails became very soft and thin. My teeth were affected. My bones ached like toothache. I walked stiffly and felt weak. I became dyslexic, and had terrible memory loss. I could not hold a conversation, and felt unable to live a normal life. By the time I was on 100 mcgs. I began to feel better, but had 'hot heads' and poor adrenal function. It was only when I had been on natural thyroid for a month that I felt life was once again worth living. Indeed because Thyroxine is not food state most people may be toxic to it. The allergy testing route shows this quite clearly. Many additives are put into thyroid medication – in Armour (titanium white paint), and Thyroxine, lactose, maize, wheat and even e-numbers can be added. Why any pharmaceutical company would want to add lactose, which many people are allergic to, is failing in common sense.

## PARATHYROIDS

These, (usually) four kidney shaped glands regulate the calcium levels in the body and are located behind the thyroid. Parathyroid hormone (PTH) acts upon the kidneys, intestine and bone tissue.

It promotes calcium absorption in the intestine, demineralization of bone, and excretes excess phosphorous via the kidneys. The level of PTH is controlled by the level of calcium in the blood. Acid foods, cola and fizzy drinks, fruits and sugars all affect this hormone. If there is not enough calcium in the blood to make bones, activate hormones and cell function then it will be taken out of the bones. Shortage of calcium is one of the worst things we do to ourselves. If you are unconvinced about coke and cola poisoning pop a piece of bone into a cup of it and see for yourselves. The pH of coke is 2.8 - which is just slightly above acid.

Calcitonin is secreted by the thyroid itself and has the opposite effect of PTH, i.e. it inhibits absorption of calcium.

The problem with taking thyroid supplementation is that this vital regulation is lost because the TSH is downgraded. The result is rotting bones if you like. It is imperative to take food state calcium such as sea calcium, which is calcified seaweed or coral calcium, which is, ground coral from Japan. Also you cannot metabolise calcium without Vitamin D. Spending two hours or at least half an hour each day, outside at lunchtime is a good way of stimulating both thyroid and other hormones, especially calcitonin. Many people who take pharmaceutical thyroid have problems with bones, especially their hips and knees.

Got aching knees?  You may need T3.  Are your nails ridged?  Do have a calcium check and or bone density test.

## ADRENAL GLANDS

These two glands sit astride the kidneys hat-like. They are contained in a capsule and have an inner and outer area called the cortex and medulla.  They keep you alive.

The adrenal cortex forms the outer part of the capsule, and makes the steroid hormones. Although ALL hormones made from the adrenals are steroids, (including oestrogen), the ones we commonly know are cortisol and hydrocortisone. Yet oestrogen, progesterone, cholesterol etc. are all steroids.

Cells of the cortex have high cholesterol and vitamin C content.  The adrenals survive on asorbic acid, (Vitamin C); this should give you a big pointer to those foods you need to eat.   All adrenal hormones, in fact all hormones are made from cholesterol.  More about how to protect the adrenals is featured in the book "Primitive Healing".

Gastric juices, saliva and sweating are controlled by the cortex. Cortisol elevates blood sugar levels, hence the hypothyroidism/adrenal connection, (HPA). The cortex interacts with the hypothalmus to control body functions.

The cortex influences the release of the brain hormones, including ACTH. Many people wonder why they feel better in the morning or evening. The answer is in these steroid hormones. For example ACTH is at it's highest in the morning, like testosterone. This in turn stimulates the thyroid.

*This is a good reason never to have a blood test in the morning. Morning blood tests have two failings, one is that the patient may have taken their thyroid meds recently and the other is that most hormones are at their highest in the morning. Plus the patient may be stressed from rush hour traffic, white coat syndrome etc.*

Allergies indicate that the adrenals may not be functioning correctly; these can also be parasites and low DHEA.

The adrenal medulla are controlled by the sympathetic nervous system. The reaction of the fight or flight response comes from these. The thyroid stimulates the para-sympathetic nervous system and this must be in balance with the sympathetic nervous system.

Long-term stress depletes the adrenals and eventually they short-circuit the stress response, and in some cases atrophy, (shrink). This is called the "Ring of Fire".

If your adrenals aren't working properly you may have secondary hypothyroidism, for which you will rarely, if ever, be tested. It doesn't matter how much thyroid is in your system it needs cortisol to make it work. (Secondary being failure from another source).

Cholesterol is the starting block for all adrenal hormones. Cholesterol then changes into pregnenolone, which in turn forms two routes or pathways through the adrenal glands. One route makes natural progesterone and stress hormones. The other route makes oestrogen, oestrol and testosterone. Pregnenolone stimulates the thyroid. Age also reduces these hormones. Our hormones decrease on average by 1% per year. If you have grey hair you may have low adrenals.

Both pathways are balanced by DHEA.

You know when you have low DHEA - you have fat legs and grey hair. Low DHEA usually corresponds with low growth hormone. Smokers and drinkers usually have low adrenal hormones especially DHEA. So how important is this hormone? A clue may be to tell you that the adrenals put out more of this hormone than any other. Many things interfere with DHEA production, such as prescribed medication, vitamins and supplements, stress, toxins, inadequate sunlight, trauma, sugars, infections, poor nutrition, electromagnetic fields, such as mobile phones, computers, airplanes, unnatural lighting, plus many more. DHEA is called 'The Master Hormone'.

The food you eat directly affects these two life saving glands. To keep them healthy, follow the diet at the end, and avoid all poisons such as tap water, supplements, additives etc.

## PANCREAS

The pancreas has two main cells. Alpha cells secrete the hormone glucagon and Beta cells, which produce insulin. Many hypothyroids are diabetic because the thyroid hormone is too low, and the pancreas is unable to function properly. Because it is starved of oxygen it cannot make these two important cells. The adrenal hormones need to be balanced with the thyroid hormones to help the pancreas work properly. The thyroid controls the digestive system.

Insulin plays a vital role in the metabolism of our food especially in carbohydrate, fat and protein conversion. Oestrogen stimulates the production of insulin. If you have TOO MUCH insulin you lay it down as fat. Growth hormone synthesizes insulin. When carbohydrates and sugar is eaten insulin increases. Again TOO MUCH insulin = too much fat. So cut out carbs and sugar.

Glucagon is required for the conversion of glucose.

Low thyroid = low blood sugar = low glucose = low brain function.

The question is – "Are you thirsty"?  If so take care with carbohydrates, sugars and starches.  Increase walking each day and check your temperature.

## GONADS - SEX HORMONES

The number of women who have had hysterectomies astounds me.  It is in excess of 100,000 each year.  I do not know anyone who has had a radical hysterectomy and not put on weight.

The number of men who cannot get an erection, and go on to prostate cancer is also on the increase. The low fat diet is without doubt affecting this.  The number of people who are infertile unnecessarily is a tragedy.  If we continue on the low fat diet, with low exercise, more stress and more chemicals each year what hope is there for our hormones?  Chemicals are hormone disrupters.

Our oestrogen dominant lifestyle is making us ill. Crude oil - the liquid gold of our centuries is causing more damage to our bodies than we can possibly imagine.  Oil is oestrogenic and plastic is made from oil.  Food placed in plastic becomes oestrogenic.  Petrol and diesel fumes are oestrogenic.  Our drinking water if re-circulated is highly oestrogenic.  Oestrogen has a great effect on our systems.  It downgrades growth hormone - like most steroids. We get fatter. The more carbohydrates we eat the fatter we become and so a vicious circle begins. Our western lifestyle is killing us slowly. Sperm counts are down to 5%. By 2025 B.C. it is estimated that our men will not be able to produce enough sperm. Fish and other species are changing sex because of water pollution. We are causing this. We can see the masses of rubbish that collects in plastic islands polluting our seas.

Most importantly oestrogen excess drowns the thyroid. It needs small amounts to carry it around our body. Our blood vessels and veins need a small amount of it to dilate them. Too much makes us very ill. We become fat and lethargic. It also creates hyper-insulinism, (excess of insulin). This in turn exhausts the adrenal glands, which stimulate alfa and beta pancreatic cells to multiply and release. Diabetes may be the result. If you are thirsty then you may be on your way to diabetes.

The current thinking of the medical profession is that HRT should deliver oestrogen in doses to make us well. They totally disregard that oestrogen in high doses can cause breast cancer. Also oestrogen cannot work without NATURAL progesterone. Progesterone stimulates the thyroid and makes cortisol, which interacts with the thyroid. We should be given natural progesterone, which interacts with phytooestrogens (plant oestrogens); from our food and keeps us well. Current research in the USA shows women die and have blood clots on high doses of HRT. The long-term studies on HRT in the UK and the US seem to have both been abandoned.

I have seen the slimming effect of natural progesterone. Bones return too normal, after time, (up to 2 years), although a significant rise happens after about six weeks, especially if coral calcium is added. Skin is less wrinkled and softer. Aching joints disappear. The thyroid works better with it. It stimulates the liver and keeps us healthy. It doesn't matter if you have a womb or not from the age of 35 you usually need natural progesterone - if for nothing else for your bones. It is not only oestrogen that protects bones from decline but natural progesterone. Mexican wild yam helps to balance the female hormones.

Currently women are given too high doses of HRT, which can give them cancer of the womb and many other problems. There is no need for this. Few are given testosterone, which women make naturally. Even less women are given natural progesterone. To make matters worse the pharmaceutical companies import natural progesterone - it comes from wild yams in the Philippines and Mexico- and because it is natural they cannot patient it so they take out the first twenty or so atoms and can make us very ill. This product is called progestin, although any doctor will swear it is progesterone. It can benefit us in small doses or interfere with our T3 production in the liver. Both female hormones in excess can make our stomachs too acid. Make our hair fall out. (This can be also a low DHEA problem). They can prevent our parasympathetic nervous system from working properly and cause many problems. For further details may I suggest that ALL women should read Dr. John Lees' book - "Natural Progesterone".

I have taken so many forms of HRT over a 25 year period that I feel I am able to write with knowledge about this. Do you know for example that some oestrogens are derived from horse's urine? Those horses are pregnant and can be tied up for 23 hours each day to enable the collection of this hormone. My bust went up by two inches almost overnight!

At first you feel all right on oestrogen, this is usually because you are low in it. After a couple of months things start to go wrong. By six months most women have had enough. (Roughly the time it takes the adrenals to break down). By six years the hormones from the adrenals, thyroid and endocrine system are at low points. Like me your hormone regulation may be lost. We are being turned into obese morbid's by this poor delivery of HRT. Getting the balance right often feels like an impossible task. Too little and the thyroid fails to work completely. Too much and we become depressed then thyroid does not work at all. However if natural progesterone, DHEA and pregnenolone supplements are given the body

41

regains its' natural balance.  HRT interferes with
liver function and T3 metabolism.  When you put a
hormone into the body the pituitary sends out
signals, which switch off other hormones too.

## WHAT MAKES THE THYROID BECOME ILL?

Several drugs and products of the 20th century
make our thyroids ill.  All listed interfere with the
blood tests.  These are HRT (oestrogen), Asprin,
(stops binding to the carrier protein), hair products
and medicines that contain alum, (a sulphate
mixture of aluminum and potassium).  Tap water
contains alum and some other chemicals.  Pots and
cooking utensils are often made from aluminum.
Our medications can come in aluminum.  Cough
medicines and expectorants affect the thyroid.
Caffeine is another.  Lithium is one of the many
medicines that down grades the thyroid.
Amoidarone a heart drug inhibits T4 by reducing
the binding of iodine thus reducing T3 conversion
levels - it can also cause hyPER thyroidism if given
in large doses.  Propranolol (Inderal) is a beta-
blocker - it reduces T3 levels.  Phenytonin
(Epanutin) is often used to control seizures,
epilepsy and fits interferes with the protein binding
process.  Salicylates such as Asprin and other
painkillers also bind to the proteins inhibiting full
functions of T4 to T3 conversion.  Fenclofenac
taken for rheumatic disease is well documented in
the NIMS for interfering with thyroid function tests.
Carbamazepine taken for diabetes and epilepsy has

an antidiuretic action and creates hypothyroidism. Corticosteriods are used for a wide range of illnesses from acne to rheumatic disorders. If the adrenals are not functioning correctly then they often need a short-term boost of cortisol to settle the thyroid into a working mode. Steroids however downgrade growth hormone. Take care because long term these do affect the liver adversely. Especially when prescribed in high doses.

Some of the toxic combinations people are prescribed by their doctors, or they take themselves, especially supplements, which can be of very poor quality leaves me flabbergasted. Looking back in desperation I was included in that summary. I know only too well you will try anything to feel better.

## ALPHABETICAL REFERENCE LIST
### Simple meanings

**Vitamin A** - interference of this vitamin is caused by: cortisone, alcohol, fluorescent light, air pollution, polyunsaturated fats, tinned food, frying food, nitrates, caffeine, iron, lead, oxygen, chemotherapy, antacids, antibiotics, Asprin, laxatives, some medicines.

Enhancement of vitamin A - carotines, calcium, iodine, phosphorous, zinc, choline, folic acid, vitamins: B12, C, D, E Vitamin A alleviates hyPERthyroidism and help wounds to heal. It also

43

improves function of the adrenal glands. Four ways to obtain vitamin C are: beta-carotene, oily fish and CoQ10, multivitamin tablets.

Absorb through food and not oil capsules, which are often toxic.

**Symptoms of low vitamin A** - loss of appetite, diarrhea, halitosis, blood-shot eyes, eye problems, night blindness, acne, ear problems, itchy scalp, and sinusitis.

**Acne** - healing foods are: shellfish, nuts, poultry, meat and zinc.

**Adrenal malfunction** is caused by long-term stress, (over production), pituitary failure, (whiplash), internal damage, poisons, (caffeine in large doses), drugs and chemicals, thyroid malfunction, and incorrect diet. Indicators of adrenal malfunction are: obesity, swollen stomach, thin skin, acne, diabetes, mood swings, low blood pressure illness or extreme anxiety. You may also have exhaustion and tiredness.

Cushing's disease or over production of adrenal glands may be caused by over production or overdose of cortisone, or a pituitary tumour, or an adrenal tumour.

Adrenals link up to the thyroid and the thyroid needs cortisol to make it work correctly. The adrenals are two small glands weighing around 4 grams each. Their health is vital to our well being. The medulla makes noradrenaline and adrenaline for the fight or flight response. The cortex makes our stress hormones and controls our blood pressure. It balances the glucose in our bloodstream and acts to control our blood sugar levels. The sex hormones are made in the cortex and also anabolic steroids are made here naturally. DHEA is made in the cortex and it balances the hormones and boosts the immune system. DHEA is produced more than any other hormone and it interacts with growth hormone, if DHEA is low then so is growth hormone and vice versa.

**Aluminum -** downgrades the thyroid and has been proven to contribute to poor memory and brain diseases. Throw out your aluminum cooking pots and pans and your cooking foil. People suffering from Alzheimer's disease can have high levels of this in their brains. (They also need Vitamin B12 and a high oil diet).  Coconut oil is said to improve this debilitating illness, 5 tablespoons per day.

**Vitamin B2 -** helps eye problems, facilitates metabolism of carbohydrates, vital for energy production, thyroid malfunction can be caused by deficiency of this vitamin. It alleviates - acne, carpel tunnel syndrome, cataracts, dandruff, eczema, dry lips, depression, numbness in hands and feet, absorption of iron, migraines.

Things that interfere with B2: cooking destroys it, antibiotics, alcohol, the Pill. If you have very bad migraines it is generally recommended you should take up to 400mgs per day. Microwaving destroys around 60% of all enzymes in our food.

**Beta-carotine** - protects the body from polyunsaturated fats, (free radicals). It is said to help in all cancer cases and reduces heart attacks by up to 50% and strokes by 50% at 50mgs per day.

It improves the eyes and enhances the immune system. It concentrates in the thyroid gland, liver, and heart and strengthens lungs. Iodine facilitates the conversion of it to vitamin A. Light destroys it. Smoking destroys it. If you have diabetes mellitus you may have problems converting it to vitamin A. It has a half-life of 12 days. The average daily dose is 10 - 20 mgs. If you are not allergic to carrots, (most people are not), try half a cup of carrots each day, wash peel and wash again before eating.

**Blood tests** vary from area to area, so do reference ranges. There is no British Standard. For primary hypothyroidism TSH is usually the frontline test, followed by FT4. FT3 is not usually carried out, and conversion problems rarely picked up. Tertroxin (T3, Cytomel/Cynomel), is not usually prescribed or tested for. Most doctors think that hypothyroidism is not caused by secondary failure, and because of this we are not tested for secondary failure of other endocrine glands. Reference ranges stated by thyroid specialists are: TSH 0.15 - 3.5mU/1 and FT4 10 - 25. See Blood Test Information sheets for further details. Remember to please refuse a blood test in the morning as this is when your hormone levels are at their highest. This is because sleep makes hormones. Starvation affects blood tests too; it causes reverse T3 in the liver for one. So many things affect these tests such as coffee, stress etc. You are entitled to have a copy of the results, as they are yours. You are entitled to a copy of your tests and to see your file by making an appointment to view it at your doctors. You are entitled to explanations.

**Vitamin C -** helps manufacture collagen for the skin. Collagen is the building block for cartilage, bone, tendons and muscles. It also helps with rheumatic pain. C and E reduce heart disease. The adrenals are maintained by C. It is essential for growth hormone releasing hormone. It facilitates the production of T4. It detoxifies the system. It produces collagen. It converts the blood fats LDL's to HDL's. It facilitates calcium into the system. It eliminates uric acid (sweaty toes). It prevents the oxygenation of other vitamins. Insulin transports it into the cells. Iron decreases the absorption of this vitamin. It does not remain in the body for long.

The following destroys it: antibiotics, anticoagulants, anti-convulsants, anti-depressants, anti-histamines, Aspirin, barbiturates, (including sleeping tablets), cortisone, steroids, tetracycline, alcohol, tobacco, canned foods, irradiated foods, freezing foods, pasteurization, stress. It does NOT cause kidney stones or destroy B12. The RDA is 60mgs. Arthritis sufferers should have 50 - 100 grams per day. If you are stressed and your adrenals become exhausted 15 - 25 grams per day is generally recommended. Excessive vitamin C damages DNA. Blood group 'O' should take care with supplements, increase vitamin C using food. Some supplements contain citric acid, which can be counter productive if you are blood group O, also check for sweeteners and sorbitol. Some vitamins, especially children's contain sorbitol, this should always be avoided.

**Cabbage family** - cruciferous contains chemicals called progoitrins and isothiocyanates. These interfere with iodine uptake and create goiters. They are: broccoli, cabbage, radish, turnip, sprouts, mustard, cauliflower, and spring greens. These remove oestrogen from the stomach. Broccoli has the highest vitamin content of all vegetables and because of this could be eaten sparingly, no more than once a week.

**Calcium** - care must be taken because some preparations contain lead and aluminum – coral and sea calcium are the best.

**Cholesterol** - there are two types HDL high density

lipids and LDL low density lipids. You need HDL cholesterol for all hormone production, adrenal and heart health. 35% of people die from LOW cholesterol levels. The U.K. average is 5.2, five is the right level. All hormones are made from cholesterol. Anti-cholesterol drugs are banned from most countries except the UK and the USA. In Germany 52 people died from taking these drugs. Good oils, 3 fluid ounces per day, are one of the most vitally important things you need to eat.

**Colourings** - E102, 104, 110, 162, (150 is caramel). E127 is actually iodine and now banned as a food colouring, however it can be found in imported foods such as French glace cherries and coats some prescription drugs. These are found in processed food, squash, soft drinks, jam, margarine, biscuits and cakes. They are asthma and hyperactivity triggers. Avoid.

**Doctor's advice on the thyroid** varies vastly. Some say it is like speed and you will burnout. Some say it gives you a heart attack; the opposite is true, if you have a normal heart and you take the correct amount of thyroid hormones you stand a 95% reduction of having a heart attack. (For more reading - see Dr. Broda Barnes book.) This myth came about because some physicians in the 1930's were prescribing stupid amounts of natural thyroid from 5 grains to an unbelievable 40 grains. Like everything else too much is as bad as too little. Some doctors will tell you about suppression. It is correct that Thyroxine suppresses the TSH, (thyroid stimulating hormone), and interferes with normal function which is why natural thyroid works so much better. Finally you may be told that you will develop osteoporosis, which needs careful attention. If your thyroid is working properly then you will be able to metabolize oestrogen and progesterone and if it not you probably won't. This is because the thyroid is carried around the body on the back of oestrogen.

Hypothyroidism - the percentage of hypothyroids goes by population e.g.1% of one year olds may have it, 50% of fifty year olds, 80% of eighty year olds etc. So by the time you are fifty you are said to be half way there.

**E - numbers generally** - E412, 414, 440, 460, 322, 422 are found in sauces, soups, bread, biscuits, cakes, desserts, ice cream, margarine, spreads, jam, chocolate, milk shakes. They can cause flatulence and can reduce liver performance. Avoid.

**Epilepsy** - one in four is misdiagnosed. Hypothyroidism can also trigger faints and distorted brain waves because the brain is starved of glucose and oxygen. 6,000 are misdiagnosed each year. There is no test. EEG tests are often misread or misunderstood by G.P.'s. You can lose your driving licence, and have to be seizure free for one year to get it back. The medicine is anticonvulsant, which causes short-term memory loss, balance and co-ordination problems, and often these do not show up at first. Afterwards the medicine takes two to six months to leave your system.

**Flavourings** - MSG, (monosodiumglutomate), 621, 622, 631. Found in Chinese food, gravy powders, stock cubes, and some packet soups, tinned and processed meat. MSG is a thyroid inhibitor and in large doses gives hallucinations. Avoid.

**FOOD STATE VITAMINS** - Most vitamins bought by us over the counter are pure B.P. state vitamins. All vitamins are extracted from coal and some are added to foods to be absorbed. However the dosages, additives and heavy metals that contaminate some of these products is to me, frankly astounding. Food state natural vitamins must find lipids, proteins and chelates to be absorbed. Food state vitamins are more easily absorbed. Calcium is often sold to us as calcium carbonate, which is chalk. But humans do not eat chalk. Plants that live on chalk absorb it, and it is in this state that humans can utilize it fully. Food state vitamins have their own amino acid profile. All food state vitamins are additive, preservative and yeast free. So what is the best way to get these? Buy a juicer, wash peel and wash again organic or own grown foods. Too many people overdose and poison their lymph with toxic combinations of supplements believing them to be

51

helping. Blood group O cannot take vitamin supplements for long as it can lower their energy by up to 20%.

**Folic acid** - a must for pregnant mums but it is also excellent for cell regeneration. It works on 20 different enzymes to build DNA and restores normal nerve function. Testing shows around 70% of people are short of this. If you increase your vegetables it helps.

**Genetically altered food** - 60% of imported food is genetically altered. It is said there is no soya bean that has not been genetically engineered. The humble tomato was one of the first foods know to be engineered; at the turn of the century it was inedible, until the Victorians took a hand in matters.

**Heart attacks** - thyroid therapy reduces these. 35% of heart attacks occur in people who have LOW cholesterol levels. Low HDL that is. You need HDL, (high density lipids) for normal body function. It is not cholesterol that kills, but the furring up of the arteries. Babies are born with 40 times the recommended level of cholesterol, and they don't die from it. Brains are 78% cholesterol. When an artery rips or wears cholesterol rushes to seal it – thus keeping you alive and not internally bleeding to death.

**Herbs** - Soapwort for rheumatism and itchy skin.

Sage is good for menopause. Rue for epilepsy, vertigo, clear eyesight and poisons. Periwinkle is good for diabetes and hemorrhages. Lavender is antiseptic and healing - good for hysteria, fainting, giddiness, headaches – and a good nights sleep. Lungwort for chest disorders. Lads Love for hair growth. Parsley for a sweet breath, acid tummy, kidney ailments and rheumatism. Fennel for menopause, eyesight and a neat waistline, lovely washed and juiced. Cowslip for insomnia, and wrinkles. Comfrey to heal bones. Chervil for bad breath and stomach aches. Catmint for headaches, nightmares and bruises. Lemon balm strengthens the brain and prevents baldness. Angelica for rheumatism, cold and coughs. Ginger for adrenal support. Read: "Common Herbs for Natural Health" by Juliette de Bairacli Levy.

**Iron** - usually taking supplements with food enhances their absorption because food stimulates the release of enzymes - BUT NOT IRON which should be taken on its' own, with just boiled spring water. It is important not to take vitamin E with iron because iron destroys vitamin E. Iron can inhibit thyroid function, take it three times a week on alternate afternoons with water for maintenance. A large number of people with thyroid problems also have iron deficiency problems. There are so many on the market. The important point is to look for iron that is just iron in diacalcium to harden it, without all the other rubbish that is put into supplements. It is one of the four most important supplement hypothyroids need each week.

**Lecithin –** also known as E322 is prevalent in chocolate.  It is a protein and a hormone released by fat, which travels in blood to the brain.  Lecithin means thin and the more fat you have the more lecithin is produced.  It acts on the hypothalamus where it inhibits the amount of food we eat.  It stops us from being hungry and limits energy expenditure by a signal to the hypothalamus.  It can be produced from soya so take care as soya is a thyroid inhibitor.

**Liver disorders** are caused by many things including hypothyroidism.  In fact your liver is the last to heal after thyroid therapy is commenced.  The liver performs 500 jobs and has 22 vital functions.  It removes and neutralizes all poisons from the body.  If it is not working properly then those poisons, (mucopolysacchrides), will remain in the body for a long time and a build up of these will develop under the skin.  Say for example you take a whole Asprin each day, your thyroid may not work properly because it (Asprin), binds to the carrier protein preventing it from being absorbed properly.  The Asprin will build up and your liver will not be able to remove it in waste.  The same is said for all drugs.  The liver stores glucose as glycogen and helps maintain blood sugar levels.  It manufactures proteins and breaks down amino acids, (fundamental constituents of all proteins).  It also makes bile and controls the breakdown of your food. Your liver cannot work properly without fats/oils and protein; these are triggers. When these are eaten hormones can be released from the liver and conversion can take place.

Other problems with the liver are - scar tissue, from alcoholism, and jaundice. Signs of liver damage are loss of body hair, bile problems, and yellow fatty deposits around the eyes, swollen and/or tender abdomen. Yellow or pale skin and low morning energy. Hypothyroids are usually owls with more energy at night, and hypo-adrenals are larks up and about early morning.

Helping your liver to heal requires Vitamin C, fruits, strawberries, liver (if not pregnant), fish, B12 and folic acid. Carrot and lemon drinks three times a day also help. You must cut out carbohydrates, starches, sugars, caffeine, alcohol, spicy foods and all other poisons like body products and chemicals.

**Lupus -** is an illness of the immune system. The symptoms are organ damage, headaches, muscle and joint pain, a rash over face. The generally recommended diet is: oily fish, Omega 3 oils, eggs, butter, vitamin D, calcium, carrots, lemons, poultry, sardines, and cut out caffeine and alcohol.

**Malnutrition -** is something, which many hypothyroids suffer from. It is caused by over-dieting to the point of starvation, and by eating the wrong foods.  Also at risk are the elderly and alcoholics.  Malnutrition causes mineral and amino acid deficiency. Especially calcium - symptoms are muscle weakness and backache.  Iron - symptoms are tiredness, shortness of breath, anemia, and low resistance to infections.  Magnesium weakness, cramps and muscle tremors.  Potassium - weakness, confusion, apathy, thirst, poor digestion, bloating, respiration and heart problems.  Zinc - slow wound healing, slow sex drive, poor immune system levels.  Food means feed.  Food is medicine. Your billions of cells cannot divide and reproduce each day if you have malnutrition.  Parasites can actually cause malnutrition and severe malabsorption problems.  Doing a regular full detox twice a year is important.  Some people loose their appetite because the adrenals are not working properly, which means the pituitary gland also does not work efficiently.

**Manganese** - it enhances alcohol detoxification, alleviates heart ailments, stimulates liver bile, improves pancreas function.  It enhances energy production, alleviates fatigue, improves thyroid function, accumulates in bones, improves balance, alleviates depression, helps epilepsy - improves better memory, tinnitus and vertigo.  It is good for lowering LDL levels helps depression and headaches, improves sleep.  Good for prostate disorders.
Avoid tea tannin and dairy products.

56

**Medicines** that affect the body's ability to absorb certain nutrients:
Also drugs that alter the body's ability to break down certain nutrients - any drug taken for a long time can alter absorption:
1] Antacids - they contain aluminum which also interferes with thyroid function. Long term use can cause softening of the bones,
2] Laxatives - they reduce the absorption of every type of nutrient.
3] Anticoagulants - e.g. Warfarin, taken to reduce blood clotting inhibits vitamin K. A high intake of vitamin E can cause bleeding.
4] Cholesterol controlling drugs - e.g. Cholestryane/Colestipol bind cholesterol to the intestines - interferes with iron and folic acid absorption.
5] Heart drugs - e.g. Digitoxin/Phenytoin are prescribed for irregular heartbeat (see copper), they bind to fibre.
6] Antibiotics - affect flora in the gut and often causes thrush. It upgrades the thyroid. To balance the gut eat bio yogurt and add vitamin B6.
7] Diuretics- increase kidney output. Thiazides also taken in this category reduce blood pressure but cause mineral loss.
8] The Pill - affects metabolism, calcium production, T3 conversion, the adrenals and the thyroid.
9] Non-steroidal drugs for arthritis including sulphasalizine - avoid high doses of vitamin C and increase folic acid.

10] Steroids - used as anti-inflamatories, but prolonged use causes pituitary downgrading and thyroid problems.

11] Anti-depressants - Phenelzine/translcypromine cause constriction of blood vessels, and are often prescribed by doctors as front line medication for hypothyroidism, but these medicines downgrade the thyroid and usually make the patient worse.

12] Analgesics - Asprin/painkillers reduces thyroid function and cell regeneration.

13] Anti-convulsants - epilepsy - Phenytoin/Phenobarbitone interferes with vitamin D and folate absorption.

14] Cytoxic drugs for cancer - Methotraxate can cause internal bleeding, diarrhea and interfere with cell reproduction.

**M.E.** is said to be caused by a virus. Certainly testing can show that some people who are fatigued also have high virus readings. Epstein Barr shows up frequently in research. The symptoms of M.E. and hypothyroidism are identical. In a study at Birmingham University three groups of volunteers were given blood tests. The range was 9 - 24, the test FT4. Those who tested 9-14 had severe hypothyroid symptoms. 14-16 had already had an M.E. diagnosis. 17 - 24 were feeling normal. Protein is essential for this illness as with hypothyroidism. Avoid all poisons e.g. caffeine, alcohol, vaccinations etc. Keep a diary of symptoms and food allergies. Teeth can also be the cause of this illness. Metals and root canal fillings can cause ME and CFS. Foods are one of the main culprits inhibiting the healing of M.E. Eating a low fat/oils diet make matters worse.

**Menopause and menstrual problems** (including PMS) - many hypothyroids have heavy or scant periods. PMS is common to most. Natural progesterone helps enormously. Symptoms are backache, bloated/tummy ache, headache, water retention (natural progesterone, is a natural diuretic), sore breasts, irrational behavior and moods, anxiety, depression, poor concentration and lethargy. Eat oily fish; take Omega 3 oils, vitamin D, spinach, B6, eggs, poultry, liver, lemons, and virgin olive oil. (Do be allergy tested first for these). Heavy periods may indicate low adrenal function and light periods (scant) may indicate low thyroid function. It is common to have miscarriages or be infertile because of these.

Painful periods are called dysmenorrhoea, missed periods are called amenorrhoea, heavy periods are called menorrhagia – these are related to hypothyroid and low adrenal disorders. Foods also affect adrenals and periods including PMT/PMS.

**Microbiotic diet** - is high in fibre and unsuitable for hypothyroids. It is low in protein and causes anemia. The diet is based upon Yin and Yang. Yin foods are sugar, tea, alcohol, milk, cream, yogurt, spices, and cold foods. Yang foods are more suitable to hypothyroids, Yang is hot - meat, poultry, shellfish, eggs, salt, B12, iron for the blood. D is needed for calcium absorption. People who are ill should not eat a microbiotic diet as it affects their nervous system. Whether these suit you or not depends on your blood group. (See blood group testing in "A Thyroid and Hormone Diet").

**Multi-vitamins** – contain heavy metals. People take high doses thinking they are doing themselves good when the reverse is actually true. Some combinations are toxic, (poisonous) to the individual, some cause more problems than they solve. Blood group O people cannot take them as it reduces energy levels and the adrenals. Many contain iodine, which can imbalance the thyroid, especially if the dose is at high levels. These can also keep you awake all night.

If you eat a balanced diet of vegetables, fruits, oils and proteins you should have enough vitamins for a healthy life. Exceptions to this are: calcium, iron, zinc, B6 and folic acid B12. Calcium is top of the list needed most by far.

**NATURAL THYROID – There are three different kinds. Armour** is an American pharmaceutical name, made by Forest Pharmaceuticals. Many additives are added to the dried meat to make it more medicine-like. However my personal opinion is that extensive testing of Armour shows that it is a poor grade product. If God had wanted us to have titanium paint in our bodies then I think he would have put it there naturally. Natural grain thyroid used to be available in the UK until 1985. Now we have to import it from America. More recently the FDA made changes, which meant natural thyroid porcine tablets and powder is no longer available without a prescription. (This is another aspect of the power over our lives by the pharmaceutical companies.) It is natural because it is derived from the thyroids of pigs and cows, (American to our knowledge has no BSE). 40% of Americans use Armour for hypothyroidism. There are few side effects, unless you have a pork allergy. Upon commencement TSH does not take the nosedive it does on Thyroxine. The dose can be increased easily, every four days, and it usually begins to work straight away because of the carrier proteins and T3. For those on long term Thyroxine changing to Armour and natural thyroid can change their lives. These are prescribed privately in this country, and the dose is delivered in 'grains'. A small tablet would be half a grain, taken for a week, and gradually increased until the patient achieves a level of fitness and well being where they can cope with life. I would not personally recommend ¼ grain of thyroid, as it is not an addition to your own; however Dr. Broda Barnes says he had some amazing results with this in his book. If the body has been deprived of T4 and T3 for a long period other secondary illness occur, but with time, good diet and patience, health can greatly improve in about two years of therapy. Armour can be expensive, I heard recently of someone being charges £130 for 90 half grains. Thyroxine is free on the NHS in the UK. Natural thyroid food state should cost the patient no more than £29 per month. I know which I prefer, and all others who have changed say natural it is 100% better. Remember Armour contains colour and additives. Freeze dried thyroid is more natural and cheaper and I find bovine thyroid food state is the best of all. You can order it direct but need to be tested first to see if it suits you. Glandulars are dried thyroid from animals. Some people however have a conversion problem and need T3 instead of natural thyroid. It is best to be checked for this. Jones CYTOMEL/Cynomel is the best 2 x 25mcgs per day.

**Parasympathetic nervous system** - the thyroid controls this. Upon commencement of therapy the neck ligaments and muscles change. The stiff neck and joint pain go. Stabbing pains at the bottom of your spine also go eventually. If you initially encounter slight dribbling after going to the toilet, this goes with adrenal support. It just means that the nervous system is beginning to work. The para-sympathetic nervous system affects all entrances/exits of the body, for example saliva changes. Noses begin to dry up or run more. Sneezing is common. Ears stop whistling and making strange noises, (this can be low DHEA). Ears change their range. Eyes are able to focus more easily, and light/glare is not such a problem. In my worst times my glasses all have the heaviest tint on them to block out strong light. Glands are affected by stimulation of thyroid. Saliva may be free flowing, taste should improve. The pancreas begins to work properly and insulin, (unless on HRT and a diet of high carbohydrates), is delivered at correct levels. The stabilizing of insulin means that fat begins to decline. The heart muscle is normalized. Blood vessels to the lungs become dilated, and it is easier to breathe. The liver is slightly stimulated and glycogen is released. The sex organs begin to function properly and penile erection returns. In physiological responses emotions are normal. Reactions to cold/heat should return to normal. Adrenaline and the adrenals are also stimulated back to normality – it does take time, 2 years for this to happen. Generally if working normally the parasympathetic nervous system promotes a restoration and conservation of energy, and eliminates body wastes. It interacts with the sympathetic nervous system and decline of both is common in long-term hypothyroids.

**Preservatives** - Nitrates are E249-52 found in processed meat and smoked fish. Benzoates are E249-19 found in soft drinks, beer and salad cream. Sulphates are E220-28 found in dried fruit, desiccated coconut, and relishes. Antioxidants are E300-304 found in fruit juice, jam, and tinned fruit. E320-21are also found in crisps, biscuits and pies. These E numbers are asthma triggers. Avoid. Eat fresh and be as natural as possible.

**Relaxation techniques** - yoga is the obvious recommendation because it is suitable for all ages and all levels of fitness. It exercises the internal organs as well as the outer muscles. When lying in bed start at the feet, tighten and relax, then the ankles continue until all the body has been tightened and relaxed.

Meditation techniques vary from chanting a mantra to controlled thought. One simple meditation is to concentrate on one colour e.g. blue, (this is the healing colour of the thyroid). The next thought might be the sea, imagine walking along the sea etc.

Let your thoughts flow freely through your head, if something unpleasant comes into your mind say out loud quietly "NO" and continue. Imagine a calm scene. Perhaps lying on your back looking up at a clear blue sky (blue is the most calming of colours). Breathe in slowly through your nose count to four and out through your mouth. Think soothing words like "PEACE" "LOVE" etc. chanting these quietly out loud. Use affirmations such as "I am happy", or "I am free from worry". Concentrate on your breath.

If these techniques are combined with aromatherapy the results can be very rewarding. Check your essential oil compatibility first; remember you may be toxic to it. Not all oils suit all people some are more beneficial than others. Some are yin and some are yang. You need to have the ones that heal you. Lavender is usually neutral and Tea Tree. Blood group O should avoid certain ones, especially citrus.

**Renal problems** - diminish the levels of TT4, TT3, FT4 and FT3 when measured by analogue testing procedures. Kidney, (renal) problems can be caused by low adrenals. Drink 4 – 6 large glasses of boiled spring water daily.

**Selenium** - is a mineral, it helps destroy free radicals, it protects against poisoning from heavy metals like excess copper, arsenic etc. It plays a major role in the conversion of T4 to T3. This works in tandem with vitamin E.

**Substances that enhance thyroid function** - grapefruit, glucose, cysteine, tyrosine, iodine, magnesium, manganese, kelp, zinc, vitamin A and B2. Herbs are damiana, essiac and myrrh. Sunlight lots of it, at least 15 minutes per day, chilies, ginseng and chocolate.

**Substances that are toxic to the thyroid** - MSG, Chinese food, alcohol, aluminum, lithium, cobalt, flouride, **VIP – toothpaste and tap water should not contain any**. Asprin, many medicines (listed above), bread and wheat, barbiturates e.g. smoking pot (hashish) and common street drugs. Chlorine - always avoid tap water.

**Temperature** – yours; it should be 98.4 - 6F or 36.6-8C - anything less than a degree below and you probably have problems.  One problem may be that you are not making enough blood cells for natural function. Your organs are probably also starved incorrect levels of oxygen.  The body reduces temperature to conserve energy.  When temperature is too low we get hot flushes, (US flashes), which is the body's way of warming us up. This can also be adrenals.  Take your temperature when you have a hot flush and see.  Many who are born slightly hypothyroid have short stature.  This is because of the interaction between the thyroid and growth hormone.  The body cuts off the supply to the extremities when cold and Raynards Disease is common - white fingers and chilblains.  I think we all know about cold feet.  One lady who commenced natural thyroid therapy is delighted to be able to wear tights in winter instead of thermals and trousers.

**Thyroxine** - It is commonly prescribed because it is cheap, although in recent years it has gone up more than 100% in price.  Tests for conversion to T3 are rarely done.  Thyroxine has an eight-day half-life, which means that it takes about four days to get into your system and four days to get out. Many doctors use blood tests to manage their patients instead of their symptoms, which leaves the level of Thyroxine unstable.  It is impossible to manage Thyroxine in this way because no one can detect what is happening inside a cell. The temperature test and clinical signs are the only true measure. When Thyroxine is taken is has a completely different effect on the patient. To compare it with Armour, desiccated and natural thyroid, Thyroxine does one particular job really well. If a patient has primary hypothyroidism and a high TSH level Thyroxine brings it down - usually to less than 1.5, often to 0.03. When your body does not make TSH it also does not make T3, Calcitonin, and carrier protein. The negative feedback system in your hypothalmus does not work properly, and growth hormone (GH), is downgraded because of this. So your body is surviving on T4, Thyroxine. The liver may not be working properly because growth hormone is reduced and T3 conversion becomes very low. Many people wonder why they do not feel well on Thyroxine. I hope this answers the many questions I am asked. When Thyroxine is first given the body shuts down because a welfare state has been introduced to the TSH feedback system. Most people feel terrible on low doses of Thyroxine. If their Thyroxine is not Eltroxin or Levo-thyroxine then it is a lottery to get the right dose. Many cheaper versions do exist; they usually contain wheat and e-numbers so take care. Patients report that they feel stable on Eltroxin and terrible when they are not, this is down to the manufacturer and their additives. I will never understand the compulsion to use additives to medicines as so many people react badly to them.

So what are the alternatives?  Well we have T3 – Tertroxin/Cytomel/Cynomel, which sidesteps the conversion problem.  It works very much better than Thyroxine, but is more expensive.  It is four to five times more potent and has a body life of eight hours.  Although this may differ person to person depending upon your receptors, and or liver function.  If your liver is working properly, and you have enough oils in your diet then you should be able to convert T4 to T3.  There are many medicines that interfere with this process - one being pharmaceutical HRT - and too much oestrogenic food like potatoes. However if you have long term secondary hypothyroidism, like pituitary disease or malfunction, say due to a car accident, then you may not be able to convert to T3 properly. There are few of these problems with natural thyroid as it also contains T3.

Low doses of Thyroxine are often given to the elderly.  Doctors seem to disregard the decline of TSH and think it is a supplement.  This is not true, and the practice of giving old people low doses of Thyroxine is very dangerous and life threatening. (When are we old exactly?) Does someone throw a switch upon retirement and say well you're old now? You are as old as you feel. An elderly person needs just as much T4 as a young one, but as in all cases the patient should be treated until they feel well again, the dose being stepped up at weekly intervals.  I can tell you that each and every person

I know feels awful upon commencement of T4 therapy. They often suffer poor memory, are confused. More tired than before. Find it hard to hold a conversation etc. The body shuts down because of TSH decline. This does not usually happen on natural thyroid therapy.

**Zinc -** more than half the nation is deficient in this vital mineral. You get low HDL's (high density lipids – blood fats), with deficiency. Growth and cell regeneration are impaired. Diarrhea strips the body of it. It alleviates: heartburn, male dribble/incontinence, and cancer cells. Zinc increases good cell production, and supports the immune system. Signs of zinc deficiency are: poor appetite, acne, mouth ulcers, rheumatoid arthritis, skin problems, thinning of hair, greying of hair, poor hair growth, nail deficiencies, depression, and amnesia. It accelerates the healing of wounds by 40% at 150mgs per day. It enhances adrenal function. It alleviates prostate and male infertility. It helps in reduced sexual desire.

---

**ALWAYS REMEMBER TO HAVE A LOW PILLOW IN BED AND KEEP WARM**

---

WHEN YOU START YOUR JOURNAL REMEMBER TO <u>WEIGH</u> AND <u>MEASURE</u> YOURSELF ONCE A WEEK

TAKE YOUR <u>TEMPERATURE</u> UPON WAKING AND YOUR <u>PULSE</u> LATER EACH MORNING BEFORE RISING

---

# LIVING WITH HYPOTHYROIDISM

# 2

## BY

## Susan Seymour

**FIRST PUBLISHED MAY 1999**

## AUTHORS INTERIM NOTE

When I wrote "Living with Hypothyroidism" – book
one the book evolved from questions and
conversations with so many of you.  I have
addressed further issues raised by you in this
book. A big thank you to all those who have written
to say that my story could have so easily been their
own.  I sincerely thank those hundreds of people
who kindly told me their stories.

Bionetic testing has proved to be hugely successful.
The protocol designed for each person holistically
has resulted in great improvements for most who
stick to it.  Some are impatient and don't realise
that if it has taken you years to be ill, then it may
take years to heal.  Taking thyroid and other
medication is not like taking a pill for a headache.
Cell function and multiplication take time to heal,
and the body does not change overnight.  Indeed
cell memory takes longer to change.

The objective of this book is to provide you with
details of trails and studies that have taken place
over the last 150 years.  This includes a brief
potted history of what has happened from discovery
to date with hypothyroidism - including those
factors affected by the illness, e.g. heart disease.

On a personal note I have been gladdened by the
progress made by those of you who have attended

clinics. I see weight that has fallen off, and looking ten yars younger with a new energy and optimism in most of you. My tears have been for both joy at your progress and sadness at your stories of suffering. I would say that I have learnt a lot from each and every one who has contacted me. I hope to continue to answer your questions in a caring and informative way.

Some subjects may be repeated or overlap, perhaps this will help to concentrate the memory a little.

**Below is a list of the questions routinely asked, and some simple answers.**

## COMMONEST QUESTIONS

**1.   I am taking Thyroxine – why don't I feel well?**
Answer: It is just one of the six thyroid hormones – perhaps you need all of them. You could be toxic to the Thyroxine/Synthroid dispensed for you by your pharmacy. You may have low adrenal glands and cannot metabolise the thyroid into the cells. Your diet may be wrong.

**2.   Why do my muscles and joints ache so?**
Answer: you may have secondary hypothyroidism – i.e. caused by low adrenals or something else. Your adrenal hormones may be too low. You may have low levels of Thyroxine. Your bone density may have been affected by taking Thyroxine. You may need other hormones such as natural progesterone, and without doubt calcium in natural form such as sea calcium or coral calcium. You may also need to change your diet so that

your foods are not so acid. Grains and starches are very acid and this makes the body sick.

### 3. Why am I never away from the dentist?
Answer: Thyroxine rots the bones because it stops the production of TSH, which interferes with the parathyroids that regulate bone formation and calcium levels. Try homeopathic parathyroid remedy and calcium for this problem.

### 4. Why is my weight still rising - even though I am on Thyroxine?
Answer: Your dose may be too low or it could be you are eating the wrong foods. The modern diet is actually CAUSING hypothyroidism. Not everyone can eat everything we are not clones of each other. Also if your thyroid medication is too low or incorrect your metabolism may be affected. The hormones must be balanced. Read Dr. Atkins.

### 5. Why do I have irritable bowels?
Answer: Food allergies and/or incorrect hormones. Your thyroid may be too low. Parasites, moulds, fungus, and bacteria can also cause this. Loose stools can aso mean low adrenals.

### 6. Why are my eyes gritty and sore?
Answer: You may have low adrenals or your thyroid may be too low. You may have chemical toxicity from body products.

### 7. *Why does my blood test show I have enough thyroid hormones in my blood, yet when my medication is reduced so that it is within the range I feel so ill?*
Answer: It is incorrect to treat a blood test and not a

person.  There are other hormones that make thyroid hormones work, and you may need those too.  A blood test is only a snapshot in time – five minutes later or even later in the day your thyroid could have dropped below the line.  See information sheets on "Blood Tests". It may be your adrenals that are too low causing your thyroid symptoms. Usually one falls after the other as they work together.  Some people need to be in the upper range to feel well.  I felt really ill when I was just within the range at 10, borderline, and fine when it was 20 – 23.


## THYROID HISTORY

It is important to understand how this illness was discovered, how it progressed, and where we are today.  The book encloses the latest research, time tested methods and old treatments forgotten.  The basic knowledge is simple: **IF YOUR UNDER ARM TEMPERATURE TEST IS CONSISTENTLY LESS THAN 97.8F YOU PROBABLY HAVE HYPOTHYROIDISM**. This test is a worldwide test for hypothyroidism devised over a thirty-year study by Dr. Broda Barnes.

Why is another factor that needs to be cosidered. Unless you are born with hypothyroidism – few are you have developed the condition/illness, as you grew older.  Factors include – poor diet, parasites, viruses, moulds and bacteria, antibiotics and injections, operations, shock and stress, and so the list goes on.  What we have to do is to stop treating symptoms and blood tests - and start treating causes and people holistically.

Lifelong studies have shown that hypothyroidism contributes too many other illnesses, heart disease, liver failure, cancer, strokes, lupus, anaemia, plus many others.

2,000 years ago AD Chinese doctors administered a soup of animal thyroid. The result was patients felt younger, became more alert, and were energized and rejuvenated.

Century's later Harley Street doctors fed patients with raw animal thyroid. Naturally the patients were squeamish about this and alternatives were tried. Things took another turn in extreme experimentation, and not surprisingly transplanting animal thyroid into the body resulted in death. (For both animals and patients). Of course with hindsight we now know that our bodies reject foreign tissue.

Later Dr. Murray concocted a glycerine extract of fresh animal thyroid. This did not work because the thyroid became mouldy, and did not last long. He later developed an idea that drying the fat from fresh animal glands may work, and he experimented upon a severely hypothyroid middle-aged woman. She was near death, had low heart function and severe myxedema. She had nothing to loose, (a lesson many of us should take). Within a short space of time her symptoms disappeared, she remained in excellent health for another nineteen years and died of natural causes. She did stop her medication several times but her symptoms returned until she began thyroid therapy again. For the next 100 years Dr. Murray's formula was improved upon and refined via processing en masse. This product is called natural thyroid. Unfortunately thyroid therapy then took a step back, and we got Thyroxine and Synthroid. (It is said six people in 100 need it but the majority may not).

## THYROID RESEARCH - PROGRESS TIMELINES

In 1877 one of Dr. William Ord's (of Britain) patients died. Upon her autopsy she had a grossly enlarged, low function, fibrous and mucin-logged thyroid. Her tissues were swollen. When Dr. Ord cut into what he thought was waterlogged tissues, he was suprised to find a glue-like substance, which we now call mucopolysacchrides. She had advanced artery decay; the kidney, heart, and brain arteries were particularly bad - almost entirely clogged. Six common indicators show that she had an abnormal temperature, was fatigued, depressed, had poor menses, was overweight and had frequent infections.

In 1883 a group of Harley Street physicians prepared a volumous report of 300 pages declaring that myxedema (grade one severe- hypothyroidism), was caused by low thyroid function.

In 1890 Austrian Empress Maria Theresa passed a law making it mandatory for each patient who died in hospital to have an autopsy.  In doing so she created medical progress and learning.

Tests were carried out on animals by Professor Kocher of Switzerland.  He also discovered that when patient's thyroids were removed they died quickly.  The Professor designed an operation, which consisted of removing ONLY the part of the thyroid that was swollen, and blocking the windpipe.  The patients still died.

At the same time Professor Billroth of Vienna totally removed goitres and like Kocher his patients also died.

Billroth consigned his best student to the task of discovering what happened when the thyroid was removed.  The outcome was that the arteries of the body degenerated causing poor oxygen supply to the heart.

Drs. Pick and Pineless of Vienna were able to reverse the low thyroid function by using fresh extract of thyroid and this prevented artery damage.

Eventually every day life for the hypothyroid patient improved.  A set of guidelines were drawn up for physicians and patients were diagnosed clinically, (upon signs and symptoms).

In the 1950's two important events took place in Britain. The NHS was introduced. Blood tests were also introduced. For the time being doctors continued to prescribe natural thyroid and diagnose on signs and symptoms. This was the way they had been taught, to use their eyes prick up their ears and use clinical diagnosis.

In the 1960's Glaxo introduced Thyroxine - Eltroxin. It was heralded as the most desired medication for hypothyroidism and given major marketing. Described as "Purer than natural thyroid" so that it was deemed to be better. Doctors believed that is was better and began to prescribe it. (Unfortunately our body does not respond well to pure and chemical, on the whole it much prefers food state and natural.) The fact that it was just one hormone T4 and did not replace or enhance the natural thyroid function did not seem to bother them. The thyroid test to accompany this was T4, and not as is should have been FT4 - Free T4. (In other words the amount available, unbound to anything else, for uptake by the thyroid gland).

This is just one aspect of hypothyroidism, and a small aspect at that. By 1986 natural thyroid had been taken out of the NIMS. This occurs when the pharmaceutical company producing the product are not making enough money/profit out of it and the product is withdrawn, or the patients using them have run out, due to death, GP practices etc. Dr. Barry Durrant-Peatfield would tell you that he bought the last 6 million tablets produced in the UK.

This is the current situation. Thyroxine has also changed. Many of the patients would happily tell you that Eltroxin or Levothyrxine is the most stable - i.e. is consistently the same potency. However since we joined the EEC many of our imports are of an inferior quality and are not consistently the same potency. Another step for Glaxo was to stop manufacturing T3 – (Tertroxin), this was moved to a smaller British company, and many doctors stopped prescribing that too. Subsequently T3 became more expensive and a further decline occurred - even less was prescribed. Most doctors that I know or have learnt of their actions do not prescribe T3, which has higher monthly costs. Thyroxine used to be a few pence per month – however the pharmaceutical companies have put up the price by 200% in the last few years. Jones Cynomel is by far the best T3 and it is unavailable in the UK on the NHS. Tertroxin is not as effective as Cynomel. If you are holidaying abroad, especially in Mexico, you may be able to purchase this over the counter.

The world expert in hypothyroidism was Broda Barnes, an American doctor. He conducted a thirty-year study and the Broda Barnes Institute is the world leading authority on endocrine dysfunction. Broda Barnes died in 1989, but he discovered that normal thyroid function prevents strokes and heart attacks. It also prevents chronic fatigue syndrome, cancer, premature aging, furred arteries, and many other life-threatening illnesses. He also discovered that 42% of the population will get the illness at some point in their lives. It also affects 1 in 3 women in their lifetime.

Unfortunately Dr. Barnes book is out of print in the UK, and many or most of our GP's have never read it. Dr. Stephen Langer has embraced the Barnes philosophy and taken it to new levels declaring that hormone malfunction is the root of many illnesses. I totally agree with him. His book "Solved - The Riddle of Illness" speaks volumes. Dr. Hulda Clark says that thyroid disease can be caused by mercury poisoning from the teeth. It has been proven that marijuana also affects the thyroid because it burns at a high temperature and kills the cells that way. Dr. Robert Atkins then takes this to higher levels linking food to the problem of hypothyroids. I.e. which foods should we eat to support our hormones? One step further is the excellent work done by Dr. Peter D Adamo on blood group toxicity to foods.

More recently a town in USA had a butcher who included neck meat, which had thyroid in his beef burgers – and the result? The town had an unusually slim population. The health concern was that the population were over-active in their symptoms of thyroid, racing pulse, agitation etc. When the thyroid was taken out of the meat they became like the rest of America – 40% clinically obese, (and rising).

## INDICATORS – Is it my thyroid?

Take your temperature readings if you are NOT menstruating or ovulating. So the ideal time would be the week after menstruation or the end of menstruation. Do this by shaking down a glass thermometer at night before going to sleep. When you wake up and while you are cosy and warm in bed pop the thermometer under your armpit for ten minutes, yes it does take that long. WRITE IT DOWN IN A NOTEBOOK. Also take your pulse (pottering about) for a whole minute WRITE IT DOWN. Do this for a week. Later on in the day write down your pulse again when you are pottering about – i.e. not resting and not doing aerobics, or exerting yourself. WRITE IT DOWN. By writing things down you can monitor your progress.

LOW SEX DRIVE

Many people - both sexes - loose their sex drive. This can be a death knoll to any already overstretched relationship. It is common for hypothyroids to marry each other. "He doesn't understand" is a common cry - and "I can't get an erection" is also common, sustaining it even more so.  Loss of libido can be overwhelming.  Low oxygen causes the tissues to become shrunk.  The vagina looses sensation, the person is always cold, and breasts loose their ability to become erect, menstrual pain is common - along with heavy bleeding.  Periods become frequent or the cycle is lost and becomes absent. (Heavy periods are usualy caused by low adrenals and scant periods low thyroid).  Headaches are acute, (low adrenals). Fatigue and feeling irritable - PMT - are all too common.  One long-suffering husband said his wife was only 'normal' for three days out of every month. He asked me why she had virtually permanent PMT.  My own temper was often 'hair-trigger' nearing my period, I'm sure I stretched my friends and families patience to the limit on many occasions.  Infections and bladder problems are all too common, (cranberry juice, not tablets, help). Urine dipsticks showed me that I had blood in my urine.  DHEA starvation can also be the cause.  The thyroid cannot work properly without female and male hormones.  It sits on the back of them while travelling around the blood.

PRIMARY HYPOTHYROIDISM

Our bodies circulate around 5 quarts of blood through the thyroid every hour.  T4 is iodine based, and other hormones interact with the thyroid.  The thyroid both stores and discharges ALL six thyroid hormones into the bloodstream to oxygenate the cells.  This function is regulated by TSH - the thyroid stimulating hormone. TSH is controlled by the pituitary gland located at the top of the spine in the brain stem area. The TSH works on a negative feedback system, which means that the pituitary sends a message to the hypothalamus and vice versa. That way the amount of thyroid released into the bloodstream is balanced. In primary hypothyroidism TSH is elevated - the pituitary tries to stimulate the thyroid to work and two blood tests (TSH and FT4) will show primary hypothyroidism. This means that the thyroid is not producing enough of the T4 hormone. It does not show any indication on T4 to T3 conversion or low adrenal function. However the time of the test is crucial. Morning tests simply don't work because our natural circadian (24 hour), rhythm raises our hormone levels at 7 a.m. upon waking. As the day progresses our hormones decline, especially cortisol.

My own experience typifies the flaw. Between morning and four p.m. my cortisol level was within the range, but by seven it was dangerously low. Thyroid cannot work without cortisol, they work in harmony together. When we run out (of even one) of our vital hormones our body tells us to go to sleep to make some more. Hence the exhaustion and erratic sleeping patterns. How many of you fall asleep in the chair? Some people are adrenal exhausted and never have the energy to leave the house.

## CRY FOR HELP

"Something is wrong," we cry, knowing our bodies as we do. We have the runs or constipation, headaches from hell, our hair is lank and flat to our heads, nails are soft and break or even peel easily, wounds heals slowly and spots are commonplace. Our thinking is slow, often we slur our words, spoonerisms are common, (getting words mixed up), and clarity of mind is lost along with memory. Our cells are starved of oxygen and breaking down instead of building up, we are slowly dying. Make no mistake this disease kills. So how can we make ourselves better? We finally decide to do something about it and our first stop is a trip to the doctors. We expect our GP to have the answers – unfortunately they are as much in the dark as we are. They do not get specific training in thyroid and adrenal problems.

## ACCURATE BLOOD TESTS

Our own G.P. is just that - a general practitioner. Upon reading "Trust me I'm a Doctor" I came to the conclusion that they are [1] poorly trained, [2] Poorly accredited, and [3] poorly controlled in hormones. Watching the news on television confirms my worst beliefs. I asked a specialist recently how many hours training he received in his 6 years of medical school - the answer was just one hours lecture on the endocrine system as a whole. It is obvious from the Audit Commissions findings that incompetence is commonplace; this is clearly highlighted by the Bristol Babies tragedy. It is not just restricted to our own country either. In America the Centre for Disease Control routinely sends out test specimens to 980 licensed laboratories, the results are between 8 and 25% of labs return false test results. In this country you would think that matters would be better, not so. The Audit Commission December 1998 report showed that 50%, HALF, of British laboratories yield false test results. This further came home to me when I asked a doctor is he had ever tested the authenticity of a laboratory. He replied surprisingly "Yes". He took one syringe of blood from one male patient at one time, divided it into two ampoules, (small test tubes for sending blood samples), put on different names, one being the man's own and one John Smith. He was very surprised when the test results came back differently, and not just marginally but significantly! A blood test costs £15 on average. Why don't you ask your doctor if they have done this to test the accuracy of their laboratory? You should know your blood group and rhesus. Blood group O people are predisposed to hypothyroidism.

While doing new research in 2000 I discovered freeze-dried thyroid. I also knew there was a simple way of testing pills and potions on people to see what they, as individuals, needed to make them well. Of all the half dozen plus formulas I discovered that freeze dried worked the best. For those who were tested, and started therapy the results were amazing. However food state thyroid does not suit everyone and you must be tested first. Remember not to guess at this as it can make things even worse. There is no need to guess any more. Each person's needs vary and can change as they age.

## POOR AND COMMON DIAGNOSIS

Plan your visit to the doctor. Once you have secured an appointment what may your doctor ask you? Usually what's wrong with you? This is tantamount to asking you for your personal diagnosis. Hypothyroidism is so subtle that by saying you are depressed results in you leaving with a prescription for anti-depressants. If you are not depressed it is vital that you reject these as they can often reduce thyroid function further. Anti-depressants lower thyroid function and usualy make you feel worse. Why would you want your already stretched, oxygen starved brain neurons to be further depleted? Next most common complaint is "I can't sleep" - resulting in a prescription for Tamazepam. The strange thing about Tamazepam is that you only sleep for three hours when you take it. Because it is heroin based you wake up usually alert and unable to get back to sleep. It actually makes the sleeping cycle worse not better. Heroin kills people because it lowers the breathing rate - too much of this and you die. In hypothyroidism your breathing/oxygen levels are already too low. So once again it makes us worse. If your thyroid is too low you cannot go into deep REM healing sleep, and so the cells are not repaired and you spiral downwards in health.

CHOLESTEROL

Next most common is high cholesterol. We are, as a nation, currently badly suffering from chronic cholesterolitis. The fad to lower our cholesterol because it is bad for us should have a government health warning itself. Let's look at the facts and figures. High cholesterol is a prime indicator that you have hypothyroidism. When your thyroid is working normally you simple NEVER get it. The current trend of thought is that fat makes you fat, clogs up your arteries, raises cholesterol and you die from a heart attack. None of this theory is borne out by any study. More than a decade ago $150 million was spent on a study of cholesterol by the National Institute of Health in America. The outcomes were [1] there is a link between high cholesterol and heart disease, [2] lowering of cholesterol lowers risk of heart disease, [3] the use of cholestrymanine or cholesterol lowering drugs reduces heart disease. Compare this with the 40-year study of Dr. Edward Ahrens of Rockefeller University who comments that the NIH study was financed by and a drug study, and not based upon any diets. Lets look at the facts and figures - 1 in 500 suffer from moderate cholesterol, i.e. slightly over the range 265mg/dl or higher. Those given cholesterol-controlling drugs had greatly increased risk of cancer, especially of the mouth, pharynx, intestines, and bowels. There were 73% more intestinal cancers, and 800% more deaths from those taking these drugs than those who did not, there was a 45% rise in gallstones, 22% rise in bile duct diseases, 170% complained about heartburn, there were 100% more suicides, 100% more murders, and 200% more accidents compared with those in the controlled study who did not take the drug. (All because you needed the correct thyroid therapy). A biochemist I.B. Friedland concluded from his study that thyroid controls blood fats.

130 years ago Professor of Pathology at Berlin - Rudolph Virchow concluded that blood vessels broke down long before cholesterol accumulated there. Without cholesterol the splits that develop naturally as we age would not be sealed, and we would bleed to death internally.

The much-publicised Framlingham Study of thousands of individuals failed to show that dietary cholesterol was an enemy. In fact ONLY half the people who died of heart attacks had high cholesterol. Of course the thyroid protects the heart too.

There are frequent articles in the news about studies that have been carried out and their results that are often confusing and should be ignored.

## EGGS

A decade ago the University of California fed almost 2,000 people on a variety of strength of eggs each week. Consider that each egg contains 250mg of cholesterol. The outcome was that there was no link between eating high cholesterol and high blood levels. The World Health Organisation recommends that we eat 10 eggs each week; I recommend that they are organic free range. Eggs contain lecithin vital for brain function. It helps maintain neuron function and enhances memory.

## POLYUNSATURATED FATS

Polyunsaturated fat contains hydrogen, is grey, is filled with E numbers, and is NOT good for you. An English study over a six-year period fed four hundred elderly men. Half were on a high polyunsaturated diet, all whole fats were forbidden, and the other half stayed on their usual diet, which contained six times as much saturated fat. The poly group reduced cholesterol initially then it rose to the same level as when they started. The other group remained the same. BUT there were more deaths in the poly-unsaturated group.
Hydrogenated fat can cause cancer and is toxic to us.

## HIGH FAT DIET

Many tribes in the modern world eat a diet high in

saturated fats, e.g. Somali camel herdsmen live on pints of high fat camel milk per day. The Masai tribe in Africa live entirely on meat and milk; the Polynesians eat 12 times the levels of saturated fat to us. Mongolian tribes people live on fermented horse and sheep milk and sheep meat, not a vegetable in sight. Of these groups heart attacks are almost none-existent.

In 1976 the American Medical Association reported that there was no significant relationship between how frequently the following were consumed: fat, sugar, starch, alcohol, tea. Dr. Atkins disagrees. Many of our biochemists also disagree. They argue that our food has been stripped of its nutrients from over farming the land. These are further destroyed by industrial processing and chemical toxicity from additives. Aspartame (in fizzy drinks), for example can cause pituitary stress, malfunction, and brain tumours.

In the 1930's physiologist L.M. Huxthal found that low thyroid function = high cholesterol and vice versa.

So after all these studies what is cholesterol and what does it do? We are born with 23% of our body as cholesterol. When we are pregnant our cholesterol level raises by 50%. It is a waxy, gray-yellow fat like alcohol, which does not dissolve in either water or blood. If we did not have any cholesterol we would die. In fact 35% of deaths are from LOW cholesterol. Our bodies naturally regulate the balance. Any excess exits via the bowel. If we don't have enough cholesterol our bodies synthesise it from our other food. This is another reason for not living on a starvation diet. ALL HORMONES ARE MADE FROM CHOLESTEROL. Cholesterol is he precursor to pregnenolone, the mother hormone, which means it makes the others and is a thyroid stimulant.

## CHOLESTEROL AND ADRENAL FUNCTION

Our adrenal glands are two little hats that sit atop of our kidneys. If your adrenals fail you are dead within three days. What is the composition of the adrenals? Primarily it is asorbic acid - vitamin C. Cholesterol is converted in the adrenals to hormones. These hormones are life giving and include DHEA, (the adrenals put out more of this hormone than any other), cortisol and cortisone stress hormones, oestrogen, testosterone and natural progesterone. DHEA balances these. Thyroid metabolises cholesterol. Oils and fats are vital for these glands to work properly. We cannot digest our food properly without them.

## BALANCING THE THYROID, HDL'S BY DIET

On a final note about cholesterol there are two types HDL (supposedly good) and LDL (not so good). High Density Lipids are seen to be beneficial. If you want to get the right ratio of HDL to Low

Density Lipids, (those found in furred arteries), here is how. Avoid smoking, alcohol, stress, and low thyroid function. To increase HDL levels walk for 20 minutes four times a week, increase oils to half a cup per day, (minimum of 3 fluid ounces), eat a high protein diet. Take in vitamin C, B6 and E, unless you are blood group O, (always be tested first). Vitamin C in high doses (it leaves the body daily) will protect your arteries and enhance adrenal function. Vitamin E helps circulation, and the dose is recommended at 300-400 IU (IU = international units). It is common for hypothyroids to have high LDL levels but these return too normal when the right protocol for wellness is undertaken by the patient. Carbohydrate is one factor that exhausts the body and for further reading Dr. Atkins – "The Age-defying Diet" gives more details on how hormones are affected.

DEPRESSION

Any hypothyroid will gladly tell you that their depression is quite different from a "black mood type" depression. Many tell me that they are in fact quite happy and cannot understand it. When the hypothalamus is not working properly, because of low adrenal function, it is usually because it is not being stimulated enough – and a feeling of almost falling down between the eyes, in the third eye area, occurs. One thing is certain - correct thyroid therapy cures it almost instantly. It is one of the first indicators of low thyroid function, often triggered by a shock, excessive stress over long periods, HRT, medication or an operation. Traditional tests show only 10% of those who were depressed had hypothyroidism. Yet in 90% who showed 'normal' test results they were clinically hypothyroid. Why? The answer is simple no one tested their adrenal function in the evening. When hypothyroidism is caused by low adrenal function thyroid blood tests do not show it.

I have heard some very sad and heartbreaking stories about people, who have had to endure electric shock treatments for their depression, and other harrowing stories of sectioning for insanity, to those of you have spent your days thinking your are going mad, I can certainly empathize. You are made to feel as though you ARE going mad by some doctors. Especially when the heart is under stress and you have a panic attack. An inability to cope because the brain is not getting enough oxygen is very scary. Of course electricity does alter the bodys balance – just like living next to power lines does. All life is energy. Einstein's M theory proves that all things in the world, and out of it, have their own energy and frequency.

When the blood tests were introduced in the 1950's patients were told they no longer needed thyroid, or their levels were reduced, often with catastrophic results. Depression, anxiety and discomfort became commonplace. Blood tests have caused misery for thousands over the years. What will it take for the medical profession to change their reliance of evidence-based diagnosis?

In the 1960's came the introduction of the Pill. High levels of oestrogen downgrade the thyroid, as do high doses of pharmaceutical progesterone. Depression follows. B6 and adrenal function also decrease adding to low thyroid function. Doctors commonly use Lithium to treat depression. It actually makes it worse because it enhances hypothyroidism. The Vanderbilt School of Medicine said of Lithium "goitre formation and hypothyroidism are frequent following treatment". One of my sweetest patients was placed upon Lithium for over six years for her depression. I contend if she was not well after six months another look should have occurred. The rules were laid down in the 1980's are that no one should be taking anti-depressants for more than three weeks. As it takes three weeks for the brain to adjust why bother prescribing them at all? Doctors have been told to not prescribe them for more than 6 months maximum.

DIABETES

Many people who are diabetic are also hypothyroid. For how can the pancreas work properly when cell division does not? The more HRT I took the closer I got to pre-diabetes. How did I know? Simple I was thirsty and could not stop weeing at night. My cortisol levels were at rock bottom and thyroid

94

levels subsequently were also at their lowest. I also had a pressure feeling in my right side near where I presumed my bladder to be. For those who have been pregnant that 'pressure on the bladder' feeling will be common to most. Once on thyroid replacement therapy frequent weeing is common at first as the body clears the toxins from it via the kidneys. Those on T3 – not T4 medication may experience this at a higher level as T3 is more concentrated that T4. DHEA can usually rectify this problem.

More importantly those with diabetes feel better on thyroid therapy, indeed complications are virtually erased on natural thyroid. In some cases diabetes improves to the point where it is negligible.

Signs and symptoms of diabetes are: thirst, frequent and excessive weeing - urination - unusually excessive hunger, almost constantly, acid tummy, rapid weight loss, severe itching, fatigue, weakness and of course high sugar in urine and blood samples. It is easy to detect diabetes these days by using dipsticks, which you can buy from the chemist. By dipping them into your urine you can tell by the colour chart if you have high sugar. This is caused by the breakdown of the energy conversion system. Glucose is usually transported to all cells by the blood. It is insulin, which allows the glucose to enter the cells. When insulin is in short supply the kidneys excrete it in urine. The pancreas also secretes enzymes, which balance the pH levels of the body. Often when my pH is out of sic I can tell by uric acid between my toes. Note: A high street chemist told a contact that they were not supplying dipsticks to people these days as the Dr. Atkins diet had resulted in a high demand, and a directive not to supply them to members of the public. You can order them over the Internet.

Shortage of chromium can also trigger diabetes. A diet of liver, chicken, and meat usually solves this problem. I take a huge sigh when I remember my diet of four slices of toast per day, no meat, or protein - cabbage with cheese sauce for tea. I was eating around 800 calories, which was a total disaster for my body. It is not only intake of calories that make you thin, I am living proof of that, my weight just went up and up. Doctors told me to cut down on calories and fat. What calories and fat I asked? (Funny looks ensued). It's hormones that make you fat and hormones that make you thin. But the right diet to feed you is also vital. Obviously a diet high in carbohydrates and low in protein will make you fat because carbohydrates only stay in the gut for 20 minutes. Proteins and fats feed you properly by staying in the gut for three hours or longer. In other words it takes longer to digest meat, oils etc. than bread, starches and carbohydrates.

The adrenals again play an important role in fat to energy conversion. Adrenaline - commonly known as the fight or flight hormone - increases fatty acids into the bloodstream and TURNS OFF insulin. So it follows that if you are under constant stress, for whatever reason, your pancreas will suffer. Another thing that affects the pancreas is too hot food – it destroys pancreatic juices. As we get older we need digestive enzymes to help us break down our food. Without a doubt stress contributes to obesity. Dr. Butterfield, Professor of Medicine at Guys Hospital conducted a study of three groups: juvenile, maturity-onset, and normal. Juvenile absorbed no sugar in cells. Glucose uptake was similar in both maturity-onset and plump normal people. Fat competes with muscle for insulin and fat wins. Carbohydrates are then converted into more fat. One of the few reasons overweight hypothyroids should NOT eat carbohydrates. Recommended foods are: raw fruit and vegetables from recommended list earlier in this book, part one. Nuts should be eaten with care, spinach, prunes, blackberries, and all berries, sweet potatoes, apples (washed and peeled to get rid of pesticides), raisins, pineapples, lightly cooked pears and plums. However we all should be food tested to see what foods our bodies likes and dislikes. These recommendations are only general. Each person is an individual and blanket universal protocols for living simply do not work.

Problems with obesity come largely from our western diet. Fatty sugary foods stimulate intestinal bacteria to produce oestrogen. I contend that wheat and carbohydrates are oestrogenic anyway, they are certainly acid. Potatoes and parsley definitely are oestrogenic. It is cumulative - the more wheat and starchy sugary foods that are eaten the fatter we get. Insulin also affects the amount of cholesterol deposits we have in our arteries. Insulin is made of 50 amino acids so the need for meat is even more important.

HELPING DIABETES

1]    Cut out refined sugar and ALL man made carbohydrates, (most food contains some carbs. e.g. fruit vegetables etc.)
2]    Eat chromium rich foods
3]    Avoid stress
4]    Do not smoke or drink alcohol
5]    Walk regularly, but don't overdo it, 15 minutes twice a day
6]    Eat seven portions of vegetables and/or fruit per day
7]    Avoid all chemicals; yes that includes body products and industrial make-up
8]    Avoid all preservative and additives
9]    Check your body temperature daily
10] Use dipsticks to regulate your diabetes properly
11]   Avoid fizzy drinks and cordials
12]   Be as natural as possible
13]   Yoga helps, especially the breathing exercises
14] If you wouldn't do it to a 3 year old child do not do it to yourself
15] Make all food from fresh

16] Plan carefully
17] be positive and stick to the healing protocol
18] Be patient it takes time for you to heal

## PROLONGED DIABETES AND COMPLICATIONS

Most of us know or have heard about gangrene.
It's caused by poor circulation and poor blood
supply to the limbs. I am sure all those who have
cold hands and feet easily recognise this? Those of
you have shown me your rotting nails, and poor
skin knows only too well how poor circulation
affects us. I know about gangrene because I
watched my uncle Fred die from it. I saw his
deformed body, his unusual bruises, the bloating
and the smell of rotting flesh is quite distinctive.
He had a new plastic artery put into his leg, and for
a time it worked, until his pancreas eventually also
became gangrenous too. His body was swollen not
dissimilar to hypothyroids. He had lost a third of
his eyebrows too. I still wonder if he could have
been saved by thyroid and a change of diet. We do
not know why he had diabetes - no one else in our
family has it. He had some of the signs for
hypothyroidism – bloating being another. We will
never know now. It is possible to be diabetic and
live a normal life but it takes careful planning. The
patients' lifestyle must be assessed first. This
disease is on the rise. Probably caused by
marketing brainwashing to avoid fat and eat
carbohydrates. You don't need to be a genius to
see the connection. If we look at other cultures and

their diet we must come to the same conclusion –
which is that our diet is not keeping us well at all –
just the opposite.

BLINDNESS

Another side effect of insulin is blindness, damage
to the eyes, the retina, poor eye movements, night
blindness; you can often see two black dots when
driving in the dark. All these are caused by poor
artery function - atherosclerosis. Figures provided
by the Vascular Research Foundation in California
show that 50% of those who have diabetes for 20
years will go on to develop retina deterioration.
Worse 95% of those who have diabetes for 30 years
will develop the disease.

However there is good news. Studies have shown
that with natural thyroid, large ingestion of vitamin
B and large vitamin C plus the enzyme Varidase
these eye problems in 85% can be improved
dramatically. When blindness does occur
treatment above can reverse this in some cases.
Often elevated blood pressure and cholesterol can
be major factors. Again these reduce or return to
normal when on natural thyroid. DHEA plays a
significant role in diabetes. This 'Primary
Hormone', because it is needed the most should
always be checked first.

## FOOD COOKING

One of the most common mistakes we make is in not only the cooking of our food but also the temperature at which we eat it. The Chinese say that food should be lukewarm at time of digestion, i.e. around the same temperature as our bodies. Cooking above 118 degrees F destroys the enzymes: protease for breaking down proteins, lipase for fats and amylase for carbohydrates. All the digestive glands become overworked and break down. So if you want to put life back into your pancreas eat raw food. An indicator of poor digestive function is an acid tummy. Also increase your sea/coral calcium. Always cook fried food at less than half the maximum temperature, or mark 3.

## PARASITES

The thyroid regulates the digestive system and people with thyroid problems usually have parasite levels which are <u>very high</u> – a herbal detox is recommended as a two week repeatable, (in two weeks to kill the eggs), regime. Take care to detox regularly. Every cancer cell has a parasite inside.

# Chinese Herbal Detox

Chinese Tiao He ("bring about harmony") is a gentle, yet effective herbal cleansing program, which helps, cleanse the body and promote better health. Chinese Tiao He combines Chinese and

Western herbs known to absorb toxins from the bowel, improve elimination, expel parasites and worms, detoxify the kidneys and liver, purify the blood, and cleanse the entire body of cellular wastes.

Chinese Tiao He is highly recommended for anyone beginning herbal supplement programs, before starting a fast or weight management regime, or just as a maintenance "spring cleaning."

Chinese Tiao He is beneficial for acne, allergies, body odour, constipation, dry stools, fatigue, gastrointestinal disorders, halitosis, headaches, haemorrhoids, inflammatory skin conditions, intestinal parasites/worms, lymphatic inflammation, menstrual problems, obesity, and swollen abdomen.

Chinese Tiao He comes in convenient to use packets:

1. Black Walnut Hulls capsule

Black walnut has anti-fungal and astringent properties. The active constituents in black walnut, various tannins and a quitione compound called juglone, are primarily responsible for the herb's anti-parasitic and worm-killing (anthelmintic) effects. Black walnut has been used to expel a variety of intestinal parasites, worms, and yeast. External applications of black walnut have been shown to kill ringworm, while Chinese herbalists use this herb to kill tapeworm with reported great success.

2. Burdock Root capsule

Burdock is one of the primary detoxifying agents in both Chinese and Western herbalism. Burdock is especially useful for treating conditions related to chronic toxicity, as it stimulates elimination of wastes via the colon, kidneys, and skin. Burdock is particularly well known as a blood purifier. Large amounts of burdock have been used to purify the blood and stimulate the production of mucosal fluids, while reducing toxins in the body, thus making it useful for treating allergies and respiratory congestion. Burdock is a good source of viscous fibre; helping to absorbs toxins from both the digestive and intestinal tracts. Burdock is also used to lower bowel transit time and balance intestinal flora. Research shows burdock also exhibits antibacterial and anti-fungal activity. Dandelion and burdock cordials used to be home-made fresh from the land.

3. LBS 11 is an intestinal stimulant or lower bowel- cleansing formula. This combination of herbs also aids the body in manufacturing digestive enzymes and fluids, particularly bile, as well as relaxing abdominal cramping and encouraging the growth of beneficial intestinal flora.

4.  LIV-C is a Chinese herbal combination, which helps cleanse the liver and renew healthy liver function. On an emotional level, LIVC helps reduce anger and depression, fatigue, nervous tension, and pent-up emotions. LIV-C consists of herbs which stimulate the production of digestive fluids and bile, promote peristaltic action and elimination, relax muscles cramps, and induce perspiration to cleanse toxins from the body and cool fever.

5.  Psyllium hulls, or husks, are the outer coverings of Psyllium seeds, containing the majority of the bulking mucilage. Psyllium husk is favoured over the seed germ for use as a bulk fibre laxative, since the husk swells in water to 8-14 times its dry volume. Psyllium husk acts like a colon "broom," cleansing the intestines and' absorbing toxins adhered to intestinal walls; Psyllium absorbs the toxins produced by candida yeast, which many people are very sensitive to.

6.  Special Formula is a unique combination designed to detoxify the body and strengthen the eliminative functions of' the colon, kidneys and liver. Special Formula contains herbs, which provide antiseptic, diuretic, laxative, and muscle-relaxing effects, while also stimulating the immune system and the production of digestive fluids and enzymes. Special Formula also cleanses the glands and dissolves and inhibits the growth of foreign masses such as cysts and tumours.

Some individuals may experience "healing symptoms" such as bad breath, body odours, headaches, slight nausea, etc. Such signs are an indication that the herbal cleanse is working and excessive wastes are being eliminated. Although uncomfortable at first, these symptoms typically disappear within the first 5 days and are followed by an increase in energy, alertness, and an improved sense of health and well being.

OBESITY

As I said earlier I am always totally amazed at the transformation of patients at thyroid clinics. They return for their check ups with a sparkle and vigor, which has left me speechless. One lady so reduced her tummy, and looked ten years younger that I did not recognise her. I look at my own tummy and remember the apronectomy I almost had, (reduction of the tummy area). I now know that it was not 'hereditary' as the consultant said. On thyroid therapy it has reduced by 10 inches. I know that thanks to my lovely children it will never be flat again, but people do not offer their seats to me any more, and I no longer have to buy my clothes at Mothercare. I also realise that I was seriously undernourished by over-dieting long term, and coupled with the vegetarian diet I had no hope. I read your letters about the punishing calorie restricting diets you eat. I see those of you who want to loose weight eating biscuits - happily ignoring all the advice. I get calls from those who have visited the clinics saying that they have slipped back or do not feel well.  I ask the following: What have you eaten? Have you smoked? What have you drunk? The silliness of the adult population never ceases to amaze me.  If you want to get well stick to the diet, follow all the guidelines, take your medication - don't go on a carbohydrate binge, or puff on a few cigarettes, or get drunk - your body cannot cope with these poisons and frankly you should know that you will be ill, The line: 'Well I only had ONE piece of toast for breakfast' makes me wonder if I am wasting my breath.  One bite is all it takes.  Why would anyone want to eat something that is going to reduce their thyroid and adrenal function further?  Let me explain how it works.  When you eat carbohydrate the adrenals and the pancreas discharge hormones into the stomach to breakdown the food.  That's fine but what happens when these have been discharged?  There are none left because you do not have enough to begin with.  Your body becomes tired and tells you to go to sleep to make more hormones - so by eating starches and carbohydrates you are keeping your body in a constant state of exhaustion - and I can tell you will never be well. Thirst often accompanies this.

Hollywood stars go on television publicising their books about how to stay healthy and young.  They say the same.  If you want to loose weight do not EVER eat processsed carbohydrates, never eat snack foods, do drink lots of spring water and walk.

All fruits and natural foods contain carbohydrates. Bananas are quite high in carbohydrate. One lady was eating 3 – 4 each day and could not understand why she had problems. For further reading try Dr. Atkins Age-Defying Diet. It gives an insight into hormones, their functions and how to help balance them. Dr. Atkins talks about hyper-insulinism – opposite of diabetes. He says that a diet high in processed carbohydrates creates an excess of insulin, (indicated by constant thirst at times); this is laid down as fat. He also says that it is over-eating of starchy foods that give us obesity.

---

## FOOD IS MEDICINE

## FOOD MEANS FEED

## FOOD REPLACES OUR BILLONS OF WORN OUT CELLS EACH DAY

---

The medical profession has its' own terminology that the general public frequently find hard to understand and relate to. The terms below hopefully help you to understand these in laymans terms.

# Alphabetical index of terms and explanations

**Abdomen** - a large cavity in the centre of the torso housing stomach; intestines and sexual organs.

**Acetic acid** - made from distilling wood or fruit juices. A solvent used in film, plastics, lead, Asprin, and various drugs. Used in vinegar and insecticides. The thyroid doesn't like it.

**Acetone** - induces sleep as ether or chloroform. Used in the drug Sulfanol.

**Acne** - caused by poor balance between thyroid and other glands. Often (incorrectly), treated with anti-biotics.

**Acromegaly** - a condition, which develops in adults. Bones grow unusually large. The jaw protrudes forward. Hands become spade like; it is caused by abnormalities in the pituitary gland. This can also be caused by a tumour of the pituitary gland.

**Acupuncture** - I decided to try acupuncture but sadly it did not work for me. I did enjoy the experience and the kind lady, who was highly trained, and well recommended, did her best to stimulate the healing of my liver but I felt no benefit. Her Chinese herbs did not work either which she could not understand - I suppose that when the thyroid is not working, T3 is too low and the liver cannot metabolise them along with other medicines and food. The needles do not hurt; they cannot be felt at all in most places. I felt calm a little woozy at times afterwards. I can see why some people are helped by this ancient form of treatment. The needles stimulate the energy meridians, and who knows perhaps over a longer term I may have benefited. Some people swear by it.

**Addison's disease** – is the wasting away of the adrenal glands. They can no longer produce cortisone. The entire metabolism is affected. The person becomes weak and tired. Blood pressure is usually very low. The blood looses salt and sugar. Carbohydrate metabolism is affected. Potassium increases. There is muscle wasting and loss. Digestive disturbances are common. Inability to reproduce and infertility are also part of the illness. This disease is usually caused by the following: anaesthetic, injury, tumour, cancer, tuberculosis, virus, and meningitis. Treatment is usually cortisone/cortisol and rock salt. When thyroid treatment is commenced salt craving is not unusual. Most people are salt deficient; cell salts need it to help them reproduce healthily. Salt does not cause heart problems - the opposite is true, we need a small amount because no part of our bodies makes it.

**Adrenal glands** – man, mammals, birds and animals cannot live without them. Death occurs within three days of adrenal failure. These two ductless glands sit like two little hats above the kidneys. They secrete hormones directly into the bloodstream. They interact with the thyroid and stimulate the pituitary gland and reproductive organs. They are made up of two separate parts - medulla and cortex. The medulla secretes adrenaline and it stimulates the nervous system. Aldosterone is also secreted to regulate the potassium salt (sodium) balance. All adrenal hormones are called steroids - there are thirty know ones. For further reading: Dr. John Lee "Natural Progesterone". Indicators of adrenals not working properly are: grey/white hair, (not blonde), pale skin, loss of hair, low energy, breathlessness, aching muscles, lower back pain, stabbing pains in kidney area, blood in urine, heavy or light periods, inability to have an erection, infertility, low sex drive, virilism. Low adrenals are tested simply by doing a sitting/standing blood pressure test. Your doctor can easily do this.

**Adrenaline** - made by the adrenals is the fight and flight hormone. It maintains blood pressure and heart rate. In stress over stimulation of the medulla adrenaline can be lowered and can cause exhaustion. The stress response is: faster beating heart, rise in blood pressure, and expansion of the lungs, release of stored sugar in the liver. Low adrenals and hypothyroidism interferes with this.

**Albumin** - is a protein common in plants and animals.  Blood plasma has 50%, which is responsible for maintaining solution balance in the blood.  Found in egg whites.

**Alchemy** - a combination of chemistry and magic.  Alchemists tried to change common metals, usually by trial and more often error.  Guessing at medication is alchemy.

**Alcohol** - there are two types, wood, and grain.  Wood is methyl and very poisonous causing blindness - one such is formaldehyde.  Grain is mixed with yeast (both unhealthy for hypothyroids); beer and spirits should be avoided.  Ethyl alcohol is used in anaesthetic, ether as a steriliser and solvent.  Other alcohols are: varnish, lacquer, adhesive, and glycerine, preservatives used in food, inks, and explosives.  A suggestion to all DIY-ers do please use a mask, and have high ventilation.  Alcohol also lowers adrenal response and liver function, and depresses the immune system.  It causes the platelets in our blood to become sticky and it reduces the lungs capacity to carry oxygen.  It makes arthritis worse.  Breathing pure oxygen causes arthritis pain to decrease.  I have noticed that pains in my knee joints have improved since going on natural thyroid.

**Allergy** – can be caused by variations in blood groups and low adrenal function.  The more allergies you have is an indicator of low adrenal function. The body identifies them as foreign objects and makes antigens to fight them. These show up on our urine. Wheat is common. Histamine is made from the adrenals and often we also make antibodies. Common allergies are: food, tablets, animals, water, drink, and pollutants. These manifest themselves as: hay fever, asthma, skin rashes, hives, stomach pains, flu-like symptoms, poor bowels, breathlessness, and exhaustion. It is recommended that you get allergy tested, your local health shop may be able to help.

**Alum** - any of the salts of aluminium. Found in drinking water, shampoos, hair products, paper products. Also the atmosphere around aluminium processing factories is highly polluted; this adversely affects the thyroid.

**Aluminium** - used for food storage such as foil wrapped items. It is often used in cooking utensils. Many of us have it in our teeth. It inhibits thyroid function. Throw out those cooking pots, trays and the foil. Don't wear deodorant. Take care with body products. Don't take medicines wrapped in this as they are contaminated by it. It can cause Alzheimer's. Lots of body products, face creams, and such like contain this.

**Amino acids** - these are the chemical building blocks of proteins, made by both plants and animals. All amino acids contain: nitrogen, carbon, oxygen, and hydrogen. Some also contain sulphur. Our genes have a blueprint for the order of amino acids making up an individual plant or animal. They are a vital part of us. Other plants and animals have a similar or common amino acid make up. Some are essential because they must be supplied in our food. We cannot make them ourselves. These building blocks are needed to heal our bodies. When broken down they produce the waste by-product ammonia. This material is produced by the cell is poisonous and must be removed by the urea (wee-in). If the process is not working properly because of cell starvation then the ammonia remains in the body.

**Anatomy** - the structure of the body. The body can be thought of as a package containing many parts, natural to each of us. Although the basic structure is usually similar we have various differences, which make us individuals. These are blood grouping, genes etc. Billions of cells make us, they are wrapped together in tissues, these tissues work together and can protect organs, help them grow and be healthy by using oxygen and other factors. Hypothyroidism starves these cells of this process. Cell, tissue, and organ damage may result. It takes about two years for our cells to repair themselves through thyroid medication that is working and metabolising.

**Androgens** - hormones that give male appearance - like testosterone. They are steroids and are made

113

by both sexes, the female to a lesser degree.  We all need these.

**Anaemia** - caused by lack of haemoglobin in the blood.  Haemoglobin is a red protein that carries oxygen around the body.  Hypothyroids are usually dangerously below the limit.  Haemoglobin carries oxygen to the cells and the red cell level is too low in anaemia.  The outcome of this is often a pale complexion, shortness of breath, weakness, a sluggish brain, and low T cells resulting in a low immune system.  Anaemia lowers the body's resistance to other diseases.  There are three types of anaemia - loss of blood, destruction of red blood cells, defective blood clotting.  These are caused by haemorrhage, genetics, infectious bacteria, virus, parasites, or scarlet fever.  Snakebite is fairly rare in the UK, but it is a contributing factor.  We can help by eating the right diet, taking iron (on its own with spring water), eating liver (unless pregnant), taking B12, and avoiding radiation. Anaemia can cause baldness, or thinning hair.  This condition is very common in hypothyroids - virtually everyone in later life needs help with their iron.

**Anaesthetics** - are substances, which affect the nerves.  They cause loss of feeling and consciousness.  They reduce or eliminate reflex activity and relax muscles.  There are two types, general and local.  General is used for complete loss of consciousness.  Some are given by inhalation; the patient inhales volatile chemicals

114

such as ether, nitrous oxide, ethylene; cyclopropane or chloroform. If you are having an operation try to avoid chloroform based anaesthetics, as they can cause liver damage. Any anaesthetic can cause adrenal and pituitary damage. Non-volatile ones are usually given intravenously. Local are used to numb a particular part of the body and the patient is usually conscious. Novacain is used by dentists. Hypothyroids can't cope with anaesthetics and many feel very much worse after surgery. Irreparable damage to adrenal cells is common. Pituitary haemorrhage is also common. Please try to avoid whenever possible.

**Blood groups** - Unless you have either had a blood transfusion, given blood, had an operation or a baby it is unlikely that you would know what your blood group type is.

You may think that blood groups are insignificant in hypothyroidism or any other illness - this is not so. Certain blood groups are affiliated with certain illnesses. For example group O is the oldest in the world. These people were hunter gathers and lived on animals and fruits/vegetables. As the world began to develop A came along and animal husbandry became common along with agriculture. They were the first farmers so to speak. Their digestive tracts and immune systems also changed to this new diet. Then group B evolved in the plains of Russia where animals and dairy products were the dominant part of the diet.  AB is a modern blood group – its' found in less than 5% of the population but is the most adapted to the modern way of life.  This progress in mankind is reflected in the typing.  O can give to all but only receive from O.  That's why blood banks are always asking for that particular group.

Blood group O - the hunter often has an over active immune system which can attack itself.   It may also have blood clotting disorders, be prone to arthritis, have low thyroid function, can easly develop ulcers, and have allergies.  So what can diet do?  A high protein diet can strengthen all those weaknesses and reduce allergens. In order to lose weight AVOID: wheat, corn, beans, lentils, cabbage family.  Eat: meat, liver (unless pregnant), and spinach, plus fruits and vegetables. Supplements should include vitamins B, K, calcium, iodine, kelp, (or thyroid replacement for the last two). Fast walking or short-term aerobics are recommended daily.

Blood group A - the cultivator has a sensitive digestive tract, a vulnerable immune system and is prone to heart disease, diabetes, cancer, and anaemia.  A diet high in vegetables (except cabbage family), pulses seafood, and fruit is recommended. To lose weight AVOID: wheat, meat, dairy products, and beans.  Vegetables, soya, and pineapple are beneficial.  Add Vitamin B12, folic acid, C, E, and Echinacea.  Also do yoga.

116

Blood group B - the nomad has a strong immune
system, easily adapts easily to environmental
changes, and has a balanced nervous system -
although some of the group may doubt this last
point. There are few weaknesses except
autoimmune breakdown in response to viruses.
They are prone to diabetes, chronic fatigue
syndrome, lupus, and multiple sclerosis. All meats
are recommended (not processed or chicken). All
dairy products (except cheese) pulses, vegetables,
and fruit. To lose weight AVOID: wheat all grains
including corn, peanuts, and sesame seeds. Add
magnesium to your diet and low doses of ginkgo,
swimming and cycling is recommended.

Blood group AB - enigmas who are designed for our
modern way of life. They have a highly tolerant
immune system, a sensitive digestive tract, may
contract heart disease, be prone to cancer, and
anaemia. They can eat a mixed diet. To lose
weight AVOID: wheat, red meat, beans, seeds, corn.
Add tofu, seafood, dairy products, vegetables, kelp,
and pineapple to the diet. Supplements should be
Vitamin C, hawthorn and echinacea. Exercise
should be calming, cycling, and yoga.

**Breathlessness:** is one of the burdens of life. It
comes on when you least expect it and it can be
very frightening. Often the hypothalamus does not
regulate breathing fully, as it should. This can
happen after trauma like a road accident. The

head is thrown back by the whiplash and the pituitary/hypothalamus stalk can be adversley affected in some way. Breathlessness is particularly disabling in two life modes. One is when you are asleep and do not breathe properly, often waking up gasping. Another is when walking it does not have to be fast it can come on suddenly. Weather affects it, the lower the cloud and the air pressure the worse you can feel. The colder it is the lungs can restrict even more. It is one of the areas that often may not be improved by thyroid therapy.

**Faith:** It is usually a pleasure to attend meetings of faith healers, and people who are deeply spiritual in their beliefs. Angels are in most religions and believed to be a real part of our lives. Spiritual people have a special inner light and are full of hope, which radiates out from within. Many studies throughout the world show that whatever religion or God you believe in you will have a longer life. People who worship are healthier than those who are not. The person being healed or prayed for also benefits too. The bottom line is faith heals, and you should have faith not just yourself but spirituality too.

**Feet:** so many of you complain about your feet to me. Hard skin, thick toes nails, pain at ankles upon walking. The most common by far is that they are cold. I have experienced this for years and find it a joy to be able to wear only one layer on in winter these days. My toes no longer go white, nor do I have Raynard's Disease in my fingers any more. I had problems on Thyroxine but these have now mostly gone thank goodness. It is wonderful to hear stories of reduced shoe size, being able to wear shoes again after years in sandals, and of thermal socks and boots being abandoned in winter for tights and shoes.

**Hair**: Dyed your hair for years? Going a bit thin? Is your hair dull and lifeless or lank? Have you considered that the bleach is actually going via the roots down the nerve endings, down the salivary glands and into the thyroid, killing the cells there? Also alum is a standard hair product additive and also kills thyroid cells. If you let your hair grow naturally, and you are on natural thyroid it should have body, be shiny, grow normally and if you are on adrenal supplements too your hair should return to its natural colour from grey. Hair dye goes through the derma of the brain down to the saliva and thyroid glands and poisons them. We are not meant to have chemicals going into our thyroids. Hair dye can also poison the lymph system and help us to be bald. Remember if it goes on your head it goes into your brain. A natural non-perfumed soap is best for washing your hair, with rainwater.

**Homeopathy:** Many of your swear by this, and if it makes you feel better then I am pleased. I understand what is said and what works for many

119

people. This ranges from multi-concoctions to something as simple as holding part of, (say) a piece of beef against your stomach (the strong arm test in Kinesiology), to see if your body reacts to it - a test for allergies. It is not surprising that homeopathy works when you look at the enormous volumes of placebo studies that have taken place over the years, the data is not encouraging for the drug companies. Basically you have a much better chance of a speedier recovery on a placebo than the real thing. When sugar pills were dispensed they were found to be more effective than formal medication. Energetic medicine can scan the body and deliver the exact energetic/homeopathic potion to re-balance the body. Homeopathy is centuries old. How ever did we get well before the NHS? For century's plants, oils and foods were used. Many of our modern medicines (e.g. Asprin) come originally from plants. However minerals and the vital amino acids also help us heal too. Once again not everything suits everyone and homeopathy is made to gently heal you. It is said to improve cell memory. Different blood groups and rhesus balance on different dilutions and frequencies. O usually balances on 10C.

**Hypothalamus:** the regulator of correct temperature and breathing. On the correct thyroid and adrenal therapy this hormone feedback gland usually greatly improves. I had poor nerve receptor response, did not yawn, sigh, shiver, or sweat. Also I could not taste, smell, hear properly, and my eyes were much worse than they are now. My sense of smell has improved and I hope that the nerves are beginning to heal, although I realise that as it took me years to become seriously ill it will probably take me years to get better. I used to find it so strange and rare to yawn that I notice this taken for granted body action.

**Nails:** for healthy nails eat one cube of raw jelly per day. Make sure it has no E numbers in it. Take a chelated calcium supplement at night with warm milk. Make sure you have natural thyroid where possible and not synthetic, which has no calcitonin in it. 1 x 1,000mg coral calcium also helps each night.

**Osteopath:** My osteopath was an elderly gentleman with a basic knowledge of how the body is aligned and where things should be. He has helped put back my poor discs and ligaments so many times I have forgotten how many over the years, certainly into the hundreds now. I would slip discs just turning over in bed, or turning around to reverse the car, and 'crack' out one would pop out of place. For years I had excruciating pain in my neck, my shoulders, my lower back, and often between my shoulders. Why I could not understand? The thyroid stimulates the parasympathetic nervous system, controls ligament function and bone formation. It's much better these days thanks to the correct thyroid dose. If you get shoulder pains neck stiffness these signs are classic low thyroid.

121

**Rashes:** in my experience if you have psoriasis, rashes, itching of any kind, it usually means only one thing. Your liver is not working properly. A Hulda Clark detox course often works to clear these. They can be caused by parasites. A liver cleanse and detox should be undertaken at least twice a year, usually after a holiday or at the start of a new year. Many people who have rashes have a low thyroid, and many more have rashes because of Thyroxine /Synthroid. The adrenal also play a part in rashes as allergies stem from these not functioning properly. If the rashes continue over a long period of time then I suggest Chinese medicine may work for you. Also do a food elimination process – testing to see what your body likes or does not. It can also be due to other hormones being too low. It can of course be skin mites. Make sure your bed is changed regularly. Wash the mattress with a mild solution of non-bio washing powder and hot water on a regular basis, then air to dry.

**Thyroxine:** I have two trains of thought on this drug. The first is that it is better than nothing, but only when the dose is correct. Many people are given dangerously low doses. The second thought is why has it replaced the 100 times better natural thyroid? Why would anyone want to remove something that works so well and replace it with something that makes other parts of you ill? I think the easiest way of being unbiased in this

122

argument is to quote a letter from the Internet. It is in Mining Co. and reads "Dear Doctor why do I have to take Synthacin (Thyroxine) when I feel so much better on natural thyroid?" She received no reply. The outcome was that patients in America took their doctors to court saying that they were controlled by the pharmaceutical companies and not patient care. I am sad to say at the time of editing for ISBN publishing, (August 2002), Synthacin have just had their licence renewed without making any changes to their product.

What did Thyroxine do to me? At first on low doses of 50 and 75 mgs I felt hellish and frankly could not move off the sofa for three weeks. I lost my ability to think clearly, got my speaking words in mixed up, and could not write without adding or leaving out letters, I became slightly dyslexic. I expected Thyroxine to supplement my own levels of thyroid, but it did quite the reverse. By the time I was up to 100 mgs. I began to improve, and during the day until about three-ish I felt a bit better, and certainly slept better. Initially for about six months I did slowly improve as the dose increased. This improvement was down to two things [1] I self dosed - i.e. took the amount of thyroid I felt I needed, (taking care not to overdo this like a lady I know who put herself in hospital), and (knowing the risks and that it takes four days to get into and out of your system) [2] I cut down on pharmaceutical oestrogen. The result was that my body began to shrink, not in weight - but in size. I did feel thirsty at first like the private doctor said I would, but things slowly improved. (Low thyroid can cause diabetes). After about four months I did not have to sleep at 90 degrees any more, my neck pain went, but lower back pain remained. My hair and skin were better, and many people commented that my diet was working - although I was not dieting. My worthless feeling and low self esteem began to fade, my mood and depression lifted and I felt optimistic for the first time in years. I knew it would be the two years the doctor has said before my organs healed, but I did feel better.

Around 6 months things began to change again, slow improvements reflected in the journal of healing I kept on a daily basis. Around a year into treatment I noticed my nails were very thin, now pink not white - but too thin, especially my toenails, they were almost peeling away. Then I noticed my teeth were getting crumbly behind my front teeth, and I often had toothache, jaw aches, and joint pain, especially in my knees - they annoyingly gave way when walking at times, especially the left one.

In the low dose early stage I thought I would have renewed energy and be able to go hiking again. One quite disastrous day I set off for a gentle stroll, a climb of around a quarter of a mile, but well worth the view of the lake at the top of the fell. I could hardly move after a short space of time. By the time I returned home I was frightened, I did not understand what was happening to me. I could not breathe, felt worried, and did not understand what was happening. Too much too soon, I was told by the doctor. No mention of adrenal supplementation being needed at all.

Another incident also left me feeling worried. I could not have an orgasm. All I got was a burning head and very bad pain. I thought I was having a seizure. The burning feeling in my brain happened to a lesser degree when my cortisol levels fell and after exercise. What the doctor did not realise was that you have to get the cortisol and thyroid levels right. But when he tried to administer cortisol too I could not cope with the pain in my liver. Something felt not right. I knew there had to be a better solution. Then I discovered [1] natural progesterone (cortisol is made from it), and Armour, natural thyroid. Life began to improve. However all the way along it was just guesswork on the part of both doctor and me - I was a very trusting patient.

So what does Thyroxine do? Well it tells your brain to stop making TSH, and a welfare state is induced. When TSH is reduced it affects the negative feedback system in the hypothalamus. This process stops stimulation of the thyroid and TSH (unless it is primary hypothyroidism - where TSH is very high), is reduced to nil. On Thyroxine most TSH readings are 0.035, or thereabouts. So what happens to the other thyroid hormones I

125

wondered?  For about six months most people feel an improvement, and then they can begin to decline again.  The system is that they are blood tested for TSH and FT4.  Both will usually come back in the 'normal' range.  However one part of the system begins to break down very early.  Because the negative feedback system is not working growth hormone (GH), also declines and it is this hormone that governs liver function and glucose metabolism.

T4 converts to T3 - our energy hormone - in the liver.  The longer you take Thyroxine the worse this may become.  Also you are not making calcitonin - the hormone that controls calcium metabolism - so you can get problems with bones nails and teeth.  Then there is the thyroid carrier hormone that also declines.  The outcome of this is that the blood tests seem normal but as you say – 'Why do I not feel well?'  Instinctively we know that something is not right and each person is different.

### VISITING THE DOCTOR

Try not to be intiminated or full of fear.  It is helpful to plan your few minutes of doctor's time very carefully.  You can write to them before your visit enclosing a list of signs and symptoms, or you can take your list with you, along with your under arm temperature readings and pottering about pulse.  A journal of how you've been over the last month also helps to refer to.  Remember that the amount of information that sinks in will be only a few minutes, if any at all. Do you wonder why that 15% of the population are being prescribed antibiotics for something they cannot treat? You will probably know a lot more about your illness than the doctor. When he prescribes something for you, ask about the side effects or visit your local library for a look at the NIMS or National Formulary. Think about the numbers game and YOUR chances of becoming better. There is a new way of thinking in the National Health Service it's called the number needed to treat or NNT, it's about results and not patients. Ask for unbiased information and you are may be lucky to get it.

The mystery of medicine is a dark secret not only to us but to them too - alchemy is alive in our surgeries still today. It should be renamed misery of medicine in my experience. Feedback is not a doctor's best skill. Try the 'honey' (sweet) approach; tell him how happy you are with him and how you know he'll help you to get better. Few people respond positively to criticism although it is what some deserve.

Remember you have the right to a second or third opinion, but remember that faith will have been lost, along with trust when this happens. In my experience they all come out of the same egg/med school and say the same anyway, and in some cases it is all pretty much pointless. Another name for it is institutional loyalty (i.e. they all stick together - and togetherness is the name of the

127

game).

Let's look at a reasonably simple approach:
1] Have **a list** of questions and ask them - take a pen and mark them off when asked.
2] be **specific in your conversation** - instead of the doctor asking YOU what is wrong with you give him a list of signs and symptoms and ask them.
3] Ask **about tests** - write them down - get photocopies - if they do not do the test you have asked for, (and you can), go back and get it done.
4] Ask **about alternatives in treatment** - what is on offer - what will it do – how long will it work - are they any side effects - what are they.
5] Will **the treatment on offer affect every day life** - how will it and why will it.
6] Ask **will you need support from others** - if so what support - will key factors be life changing - what are they - how long will they last.

If things step up a level and you are referred to a consultant you need a different set of questions such as:

A] How long have you been in this job?
b] How many patients have you treated successfully – i.e. patient satisfaction rate
c] Have you been audited - when - what was the outcome
d] Will I need to have to have an operation - when - why - what are my chances of a complete recovery?
e] How are you a specialist - why are you - what is

128

your success rate long term
f] Have you published any research or studies?
g] Where did you do your advanced training?

Remember always that in private medicine you get
what you pay for.  Unfortunately in the UK that is
usually an NHS doctor moonlighting for a few
thousand pounds more.  My visit to the hospital
was so unsatisfactory that I went private.  The
result was I got the same doctor in our local private
hospital. The first question he asked me was "How
much can you afford to pay".  Needless to say I
knew where his loyalties lay and left in tears.

When visiting your doctor if he waves a wand of
mystery around your illness, in order to get you to
believe that he knows all and, and you know
nothing), remember Einstein's saying "Nothing is so
complex that it cannot be explained".  Sit and wait
for that explanation until it arrives.  Smile sweetly
and just wait.  If in doubt ask them to quote the
evidence upon which their diagnosis is made.  Go
armed with new up to date research, use the
Internet, and go to the library.  Read about your
illness, know about it.   Then take it with you.
Above all else remember that doctors are human,
and you are not obliged to follow their advice (i.e.
take loads of anti-depressants) – doctors are
nothing to be scared of.

A footnote on doctors is that they have the highest
death rate of the professions, many are alcoholics,

depressives or self prescribe drugs, they are most prone of all professions, (after dentists) to suicide. The BMA estimate that over 13,000 doctors are addicted to some poison or other. Does that sound like someone you can have total faith in? Look at the figures for alternative therapies. An 800% rise is recorded each year. I was helped personally by my local osteopath where the bungling of the NHS did nothing. My Grandma believed that they were the kiss of death. It's no coincidence that the death rate goes down when doctors go on strike.

## DARE

D is for decide. Make a decision to help yourself.
A is for action. Once you have all the information to our understanding and satisfaction go for it.
R is for repeat, Keep going over it until you have satisfaction. Don't give up.
E is for endevour. Be determined and know it often takes time, but stick at it.

## KEEPING A JOURNAL

Keep a journal – e.g. temperature, pulse (pottering about), foods, your signs, and symptoms, sleeping pattern, work, allergies etc. You can see a difference before and after if you do the six-week protocol.

## *EXAMPLES OF A JOURNAL*

1]   Get up, have a bath, weigh yourself once a week, before eating or drinking.

2]   After the bath and weigh in measure 10 points of your body each week – neck, upper arm, bust/chest, under bust/chest, waist belly button, widest, bum, upper thigh, above the knee, calf.

3] Once a week or daily, write down all supplements and doses you took, include medicines and vitamins. Many people take toxic doses of these.

4]   Write down your signs and symptoms on a daily basis

5]   Be specific when writing down your exercise regime, what was done, when and for how long.  Walking for 15 minutes per day in a fresh air place is recommended.

6]   Keep a daily note of under arm temperature and pottering about pulse, (not resting or aerobic).

7]   Write down on a daily basis all foods and drinks consumed.

8]   Keep note on outside influences such a work stress, family problems etc.

## USE THIS AS A GUIDE TO HEALING
## THE SIX WEEK PROTOCOL

It is important to structure your life and plan it. Decide what time you are eating each day and stick to it. What time will you retire to bed? Make sure it is the same time each night. Give your body some stability and peace of mind. During the day pace yourself, allow time to heal. Give yourself permission to relax, be a peace, and allow enough time for those things that really matter in life. Total healing comes from the body being balanced and not stressed.

**REMEMBER NO ONE CAN HEAL YOU EXCEPT YOU.** IT IS IMPORTANT FOR YOU TO CHANGE ANY NEGATIVE ATTITUDE TO TRANSFERING THE POWER OF YOUR HEALING TO OTHERS – YOU MUST TAKE RESPONSIBILITY FOR YOUR ILLNESS. YOU WERE THE ONE WHO MADE YOURSELF ILL; YOU MUST BE THE ONE TO MAKE YOURSELF BETTER.

## Addresses, Books and Websites

Information for importing food state natural thyroid is available.

For help with doctor's telephone: The Patients Association, on 0171- 242 - 3460

For your nearest recommended acupuncturist write to: The Acupuncture Council, Park House 206 - 208 Latimer Rd., London W10 6RE

There is usually a local healing spiritual church in each county but for more details write to: National Federation of Healers, Old Manor Farm, Church St., Sunbury on Thames, Middlesex, TW16 6RG

## **Internet research addresses are:**

Mary Shoman: thyroid.about.com
For general hormone information: endocrineweb.com

American Medical Ass. ama-assn.org/sci-pubs/pubsrch.htm

American Pharmacy sells online hormones and drugs - type in Armour in search
OR ncbi.nlm.nih.gov/PubMed/

Bandolier will access publications for you and narrow them down at jr2.ox.ac.uk/Bandolier/

The Lancet is on line at: lancet.com

The Thyroid Society: the-thyroid-society.org

Dr. John Lowe: drlowe.com  (T3 expert)

Natural balanced protocols for self healing: angelhealth.co.uk

A THYROID GLAND IS SHAPED JUST LIKE A
BUTTERFLY – treat it gently

```
┌─────────────────────────────────────────────┐
│     READ, STUDY, AND LEARN ABOUT YOUR        │
│   ILLNESS YOU CAN NEVER KNOW ENOUGH          │
│                                               │
│     UNDERSTANDING IS THE FIRST STEP TO       │
│                 HEALING                       │
└─────────────────────────────────────────────┘
```

It is essential to read about your condition and the recommended reading list is as follows:

"Age-Defying Diet Revolution" Dr. Robert Atkins ISBN # 0-09-182547-4 Dr. Robert Atkins diet range of books are available from your local bookshop, and on Amazon.

"Coping with Thyroid Disorders" Dr. Joan Gomez ISBN no: 0-85969-687-1

"Hypothyroidism - the Unsuspected Illness" Broda Barnes ISBN no: 0-690-01029X available from the British Library there ay be a charge for this or by mail order from America. (See Amazon Books).

"Living Well With Hypothyroidism" by Mary Shomon ISBN 0-380-80898-6

"Natural Progesterone" Dr. John Lee

"Solved The Riddle of Illness" (this book is an excellent overall view of thyroid problems), by Stephen Langer ISBN - 0-87983-667-9 available via mail order either on the Internet or from Keats publishing - NTC Contemporary Group telephone on: 001 - 800 - 323 – 4900

"Tears behind Closed Doors", Diana Holmes ISBN no: 1-86033-908-5

"The Eat Right Diet", (blood group diet), by Dr. Peter D'Adamo - ISBN 0-7126-7784-4

"The Pritikin Programme" (for diabetes), by Dr. Nathan Pritikin - ISBN 0-553-21034-4

"Tired of Being Tired" (Adrenal burnout), by Dr. Jesse Lynn Hanley and Nancy Deville ISBN 0-7181-4528-3

Trust Me I'm a Doctor" a consumer's guide to how the system works, by Dr. Phil Hammons and Michael Mosely - ISBN 1-900512-60-2

"Why Am I So Tired?" (An up to date look at some of the causes of hypothyroidism), by Martin Budd ND DO – ISBN 0-7225-3942-8

Self help books by Susan Seymour on Amazon and e-books

Below are information sheets for you to use.

# GENERAL OVERVIEW SUMMARY

Each thyroid suffer is different, some have become hypothyroid because of the medication they take. Anti-depressants, tranquillisers, HRT, foods and many other drugs cause a downturn in thyroid function. With some it's shock or trauma or loss. Prolonged stress of any type can be the trigger. Adrenal and pituitary failure may also be the cause – this is secondary hypothyroidism.

Some people are not correctly diagnosed due to the variations in the blood tests. The blood test itself is not carved in stone, they test for primary hypothyroidism and not secondary. Your hormones are at their highest levels in the morning and, any tests should be done after 1 pm. Doctors are advised to use clinical diagnosis and not rely solely on blood tests. The reason for this is that various things change the blood test. The stress response to having a needle stuck in your arm being one; starvation is another, Always eat A MEAL before having a blood test.

A SIMPLE TEST you can do yourself is to take your temperature before rising, if it is a degree below or more normal then you may be hypothyroid. Shake it down the night before and place it under your armpit for ten minutes before rising, if it is under 97.8 you may be hypothyroid. Your pottering around pulse should be around 80 beats per minute; a lowered pulse rate may also be a sign of hypothyroidism.  Resting pulse varies. Keep a diary of these and your symptoms.  It also helps to keep a note of what you eat and measure yourself weekly.

*Diet plays a large part in the illness.  It is important to be allergy AND intolerance food tested.  The best thing you can do for your health is to follow a simple protocol:*

1.    *Be tested for good foods for you*
2.    *Do a full month detox first*
3.    *Design a diet from fresh foods that is best for you - from the testing*
4.    *Treat yourself as though you are a 3 year old child*
5.    *Be informed about chemicals and the damage they cause to us*
6.    *Have knowledge about your illness*
7.    *Learn what works best and apply it*
8.    *Be strong and not swayed by others*
9.    *Exercise, even if its in the bath or in bed Build up to 1,000 exercises per day*

Carbohydrates are difficult to metabolise and have an anti-thyroid effect, due to the reaction of growth hormone, and insulin, carbohydrates stimulate insulin production an excess can create hyper-insulinism, which in turn can make us fat. Research shows that carbohydrates stay in the gut for a shorter time than fat, around 20 minutes; then we feel hungry again. All hormones are made

137

from cholesterol, which is a steroid hormone itself, and from which **all** adrenal hormones are made. However there is good and bad cholesterol, so try virgin olive oil and butter instead of other fats. Research shows that olive oil is beneficial; it is also a plant oestrogen, (phytoestrogen). The cabbage family must be avoided at all costs, it contains chemicals that are progoitrins (make goiters), this includes sprouts, cauliflower, turnip, all spring greens, mustard etc. – but ordinary flat leaf lettuce is usually fine for most people. Take care with citrus, lemons are best and are good for liver function also as an antioxidant. Grapefruit and oranges can affect medicines and vitamins. They can also reduce absorption. Blood group O's should avoid these. Avoid tea, coffee, smoking, alcohol and caffeine as this often downgrades the adrenals, which interact with the thyroid. Chocolate and curry stimulate the thyroid, Green and Blacks (73% cocoa solids) organic chocolate is the only recommended one. Hypothyroids are unable to digest wheat effectively as there is often a growth hormone and cortisol reduction.

The "A Thyroid and Hormone Diet" book, and the Atkins Diet plus your individual healing protocol should really get to the root of any problems, and **help you to heal yourself**. **No one else can do this** it is up to you to learn what works for you. This regime is for life and <u>you should be tested for food intolerances</u> – no everyone can eat everything. It is easy to tell which blood group you are from your food intolerances. The body has two reactions to food; it either makes enzymes to break it down or makes histamine for an adverse reaction. Foods are <u>one of the main causes</u> of hypothyroidism, remember food means feed and is medicine for our bodies.

More women than men suffer from this condition. Two female hormones oestrogen and progesterone play a part. The thyroid needs a small amount of oestrogen to make it work. It is proven pharmaceutical HRT distorts the blood test results because the thyroid hormone sits on the back of oestrogen. However too much causes the thyroid to drown and has an opposing effect - unlike progesterone (<u>natural</u> - not mexy or Provera), which stimulates the thyroid and liver function. Progesterone cream, and Cyclogest pessaries stimulate the thyroid and prevent osteoporosis. Testosterone also has thyroid stimulating properties. Women have around 10% testosterone and men have about 10% oestrogen. Pregnenolone stimulates the thyroid and has an anti-ageing effect. It also improves memory. It declines with age, as do all hormones.

There are more than six kinds of medication available for this condition. I used to take Thyroxine, but didn't feel well on this, plus it rotted my teeth, as it does not contain the parathyroid hormone. (FEELING ILL ON THYROXINE IS ONE OF THE MOST COMMON COMPLAINTS), along with doctors prescribing anti-depressants – these make the thyroid sufferer worse). Change to a food state PURE NATURAL DRIED thyroid extract, which has contains all the thyroid hormones, whereas Thyroxine only has one - T4, (this means it has four ears of iodine). On a scale of one to ten I would give Thyroxine 5, (as long as it has no additives) better than nothing - and natural a ten, bovine is best. Some people actually need T3, and not T4 but this is not usually blood tested. If you are a drinker and take other pharmaceuticals it may be T3 that is the problem.

There is also a homeopathic remedy. I find that by using this it balances the thyroid and any side effects are much reduced. Details on how to import natural thyroid are available.

Energetic bio-scanning shows only 6 in 100 balance on Thyroxine, most probably because it is not a food state. The body recognises food state supplements, and these are said to be 6 times more effective than pharmaceutical. Your Thyroxine should be Levo-thyroxine and should NOT contain ANY additives especially e-numbers, maize and lactose – these inactive ingredients can make people ill. By EEC law your Thyroxine MUST come in blister packs with the ingredients enclosed. Beware of cheap imitations, which are dispensed in brown bottles. This is very important. Remember if your adrenal levels are too low you will never be able to metabolise thyroid into the cells, as it needs other hormones to do this.

## AFFILIATED DISEASES

Aching and wasting muscles;
Alzheimer's disease;
Chronic Fatigue Syndrome (CFS);
Dementia;
Depression;
Diabetes;
Digestive and Colon cancer;
Eye disease;
Heart problems;
High blood pressure;
High cholesterol;
Infertility;
Insanity;
Liver cancer;
Lupus;
Other cancers;
Problems with joints teeth and bones;
Hysterectomy;
SAD;
Weight problems;
Wilsons (T3) Disease;

I hope the above do not apply to you, but even with Thyroxine they can, the dose can be incorrect and the strength within the tablets themselves varies per manufacturer, plus the taking of Thyroxine induces a welfare state upon the thyroid and TSH (thyroid stimulating hormone) decreases. The average level of T4 for an adult is 125mgs. This level just covers you and **150mgs is the commonly prescribed dose**. Some people are unable to utilise Thyroxine effectively, indeed may be toxic to it, and may need T3 - Tertroxin instead. Or with some they do not have enough carrier protein, or perhaps cortisol levels are too low - this usually happens after lunch - we simply run out. Taking thyroid tablets also affects bone density – within two years this has dramatically reduced and you need to take sea calcium, which is calcified food state seaweed. The reduction is TSH also reduces the parathyroids, which control the calcium into our bones. **Thyroxine is NOT a supplement** to your thyroid hormones. Some brands of Thyroxine can also contain wheat and additives. Armour is also not pure - it has a base filler and colour added. Synthacin a brand of Thyroxine was withdrawn in USA. The patients took them to court because the medication made them feel unwell. The licence was renewed unchanged in 2002. Synthacin contains additives.

Remember to **always check for additives**. Thyroxine takes three to four days to get into your system and T3, Tertroxin or Cytomel takes 20 minutes. They do different things. T3 is the energy one. Thyroxine is only T4. If you have poor liver function, due to alcohol, you may not be able to convert T4 into T3.

The objecives of the book is to give a general day-to-day guide on diet, vitamins and minerals, drugs which interact poorly etc. and other illnesses linked to hypothyroidism. The book is based upon up to date research and input from fellow sufferers. We have discovered that many vitamins and supplements are poor quality, low dosage and expensive. All vitamins are made from coal, and carry heavy metals, which can go through the blood brain barrier. Blood group O should take care with vitamins and supplements. We have introduced a mail order service. The products will be as pure as possible, as organic as possible, and at reasonable prices.

Computerised health screening is highly recommended. Using hair sample analysis it is possible to check your thyroid and other hormones. It is painless, none intrusive and easy to do. Do you have food or other allergies or intolerances (they are not the same)? What parts of you are most stressed? Do your teeth cause the problem? Dead teeth in the mouth and root canal fillings can cause hypothyroidism. Remember the word disease comes from the body not being at ease.

Not every medication suits every person. We are individuals in our make up and lives. What may suit one person often does not suit another. Finding the right balance is something you need to do to eliminate the guesswork. Once you know what your body likes, and what to avoid life becomes much easier. The modern lifestyle is often the primary cause of this illness, especially for blood group O people whose genes are used to a much simpler lifestyle.

Another aspect of thyroid problems is that we are generally much too toxic. This toxicity comes from moulds, fungus, bacteria, parasites, food additives and body products. One of the functions of the thyroid is to remove toxins from our bodies via our lymph glands and kidneys. If you have low thyroid then this process can also be reduced. Low thyroid can mean low liver function which means medicines can remain in our bodies unchanged.

Deodorant and other body products really make us more toxic than we know. The aluminum in deodorant affects the thyroid. If it goes <u>onto</u> us then it goes **into** us. **Hair dye** is one of the MOST toxic things to the thyroid; it drains directly down into the thyroid via the lymph glands.

Take care with Asprin, (this stops the binding of the protein and thyroid), and other over the counter medicines.

A new book about healing the thyroid tells about general household and everyday items that poison us. The EEC had drawn up legislation for these products. Hair dye and pesticides are near the top of the list. You can get natural hair dye.

Many people who are ill show high levels of parasites in their gut. These eventually get out of control. They can leak through the intestine wall and get into the blood stream. Each cancer cell has a parasite. Animals living in your home are a quick way to get these creatures. Grain mould is another food additive you really do not want to have as each time you eat grains, carbohydrates, yeast and sugar it multiplies, along with candida. Tuna parasites, turkey and beef are most common. The rate that aspergillus is growing is showing concern, this can be inhaled. You really do not know what is going on in your body.

## THYROID FUNCTION TESTS

Many people do not question the outcome of thyroid blood tests or ask for a copy, which they are entitled to, they are YOUR tests. Patients cannot understand why these tests do not work. No one tells them that because the T4 level in their blood is within the range, (set decades ago) does not mean that they will be well. Thyroid needs other hormones to make it work. Many people are toxic to Thyroxine and feel very ill when taking it; Thyroxine has additives, maize, and e-numbers added in some of the cheaper brands. Some doctors and endocrinologists seem to think Thyroxine is a supplement to the person's own thyroid. This simply is not true because the brain says that it does not need to make TSH, (thyroid stimulating hormone), any more and shuts this hormone down.  Low levels of Thyroxine are dangerous, and should always be questioned. You MUST by European legislation receive ANY medicine from your pharmacy in blister packs, which MUST include the ingredients <u>both active and **inactive**</u>.  You have the right to insist that your medicine is additive free. You have the right to reject brown bottles, as they are now obsolete.

Many people cannot convert T4 into T3 because of low liver function.  HRT and alcohol may cause this downturn, and many women become hypothyroid when taking pharmaceutical HRT, which also affects T4 to T3 conversion in the liver.  G.P.'s rarely prescribe T3 because it is more expensive, another name for T3 is Cytomel or Cynomel, (Jones is the very best), and this is available by overseas mail order.

Diet is 50% the cause of low thyroid function.  If a person does not eat the right food on a regular basis, this can cause the person to become extremely ill.  The cabbage family contains chemicals called pro-goitrins which means – causes goitres i.e. makes the thyroid swell and reduces function.  Starvation and excess of carbohydrates also affect thyroid function.  Fats are needed – all cells contain them, hormones are made from them. Proteins are needed for normal cell production. The thyroid cell is made from 95% protein. Your hair is also 95% protein. Vegetarianism is one of the quickest routes to hypothyroidism. For more read

'A Thyroid and Hormone Diet'. You should also eat for your right blood group. The body has two responses to food it either [a] makes enzymes to break it down or [b] makes histamine for an allergic/intolerant reaction. Most people with thyroid problems have their illness based in foods and parasites/moulds/bacteria.

**Remember food means feed and it is medicine to the body to heal and repair itself.** Ask yourself which part of your body is the same as wheat.

We are all different, what suits one person will not suits another otherwise we would be clones - each person should be tested to see if their medication is working for them, to have a food check, (not everyone can eat the same things), and to have a hormone balance check. An annual body MOT is recommended. You can have this by hair sample testing; the cells in your hair are an exact replica of your body.

It is important to find out what is causing the person to be ill by non-intrusive EAV stress testing; whatever is stressed will show up clearly. Poor food types for that person will also show. Top of the list are foods, parasites and teeth in any order.

NO ONE CAN HEAL YOU EXCEPT YOU

DO NOT RELY ON ANYONES GUESSWORK TO BE WELL

147

# FLUORIDE

This dangerous chemical - more toxic than lead and only slightly less toxic than arsenic stops the thyroid from working properly and should always be avoided.

"Thyroid Gland according to the US National Research Council "several lines of information indicate an effect of fluoride exposure on thyroid function."Fluoride's potential to impair thyroid function is perhaps best illustrated by the fact that -- up until the 1970s -- European doctors used fluoride as a thyroid-suppressing **medication** for patients with HYPER-thyroidism (over-active thyroid). Fluoride was utilized because it was found to be effective at reducing the activity of the thyroid gland - even at doses as low as 2 mg/day. Today, many people living in fluoridated communities are ingesting **doses** of fluoride (1.6-6.6 mg/day) that fall within the range of doses (2 to 10 mg/day) once used by doctors to reduce thyroid activity in hyperthyroid patients.

While it may be that the thyroid in a patient with hyperthyroidism is particularly susceptible to the anti-thyroid actions of fluoride, there is concern that **current fluoride exposures** may be playing a role in the widespread incidence of HYPO-thyroidism (under-active thyroid) in the U.S.

**Hypothyrodisim**, most commonly diagnosed in women over 40, is a serious condition with a diverse range of symptoms including: fatigue, depression, weight gain, hair loss, muscle pains, increased levels of "bad" cholesterol (LDL), and heart disease..

**The drug (<u>Synthroid</u> or Thyroxine) used to treat hypothyroidism is now one of the top five prescribed drugs in the U.S.**

**As recommended by the US <u>National Research Council</u>:**
"The effects of fluoride on various aspects of endocrine function should be examined further, particularly with respect to a possible role in the development of several diseases or mental states in the United States."

Symptoms of Hypothyroidism include but are not limited to:
Morning Fatigue
Daytime Fatigue/Somnolence
Depression
Cognitive Dysfunction/Brain Fog
Cold Intolerance
Constipation
Menstrual Disorders
Musculoskeletal Pain
Fluid Retention
Hair Thinning

Thyroid dysfunction was recognized more than 100 years ago. A lack of thyroid hormone, (hypothyroidism), is more common than an excess condition, (hyperthyroidism).

The standard laboratory tests for diagnosing Thyroid Dysfunction are:

1. **Thyroid Stimulating Hormone, (TSH)**

2. **Free T4**; the pre-hormone made in the thyroid

3. **Free T3**; the active hormone converted from T4 in the thyroid and in peripheral tissues

4. **Thyroid Binding Globulin**; the transport protein that carries thyroid hormone in the blood

5. **Thyroid Antibodies**; these are proteins that are markers for autoimmune inflammation of the thyroid known as thyroiditis. This is a condition that can lead to hypothyroidism.

The Non-Conventional methods for diagnosing hypothyroidism include:

**Basal Body Temperature**: There are two schools of thought regarding Basal Body Temperature. The traditional school of thought developed by Dr. Broda Barnes advises taking the temperatures first thing in the morning. The newer school of thought developed by Dr. Dennis Wilson advises taking the temperature at intervals during the day. It's a good idea to do it both ways.

Dr. Broda Barnes method:

1. Obtain a basal thermometer. It is important to use a mercury thermometer and not a digital thermometer. Shake it down and put it by your bedside when you go to sleep.

150

2. Upon awakening and before arising place the thermometer in your axilla, (armpit) for 10 minutes. Do this for five days in a row.

3. In women, the temperature should be taken starting on the second day of menstruation. In mid cycle there is a typical rise in temperature with ovulation. In post-menopausal women and men the time of the month does not matter.

4. A normal temperature is considered to be between 97.8-98.2 degrees Fahrenheit. Temperatures below this range may suggest under activity of the thyroid.

Dr. Bruce Rind's method:

1. Use a basal thermometer. It is important to use a specialized digital thermometer.

2. The temperature is taken under the tongue, not in the axilla. The temperature is taken 3 times per day for 3 consecutive days.

3. The first temperature is taken 3 hours after arising.

4. The second temperature is taken 3 hours after the first temperature.

The third temperature is taken 3 hours after the second temperature.

It is important to take into account the under arm temperature. This measures the temperature of the external tissues, as opposed to under the tongue, which is the internal tissue reading. When a person is hypothyroid the red blood cells go to the organs (internal tissues), to keep the person alive.  It is a safety mechanism.

Dosage and Administration:

The dosage of thyroid hormones is determined by the indication and must in every case be individualized according to patient response and laboratory findings. There are wide variations in individual responses. The effects of daily thyroid reach a therapeutic maximum usually in 4 to 6 weeks.

Initial dose for myxedema is usually 30 to 180 mg daily; other hypothyroid states, 60 to 300 mg daily. Usual maintenance dose is 30 to 125 mg daily.

Note: Desiccated thyroid 60 mg is usually considered equivalent to thyroglobulin 60 mg, levothyroxine sodium (T4) 0.1 mg or liothyronine sodium (T3) 25 μg.

Pediatric Dosage: Pediatric dosage should follow the recommendations summarized in Table I. In infants with congenital hypothyroidism, therapy with full doses should be instituted as soon as the diagnosis has been made.

Adverse Reactions:

:Except in rare instances of intolerance, possibly due to the development of hypersensitivity to animal protein in whole thyroid, adverse effects are generally infrequent at physiologic doses.

Neurological: nervousness, tremors, headache, insomnia.

Cardiovascular: palpitation, tachycardia, cardiac arrhythmias, angina pectoris.

Gastrointestinal: diarrhea, abdominal cramps.

Miscellaneous: sweating, heat intolerance, fever, weight loss Estrogen, Oral Contraceptives: Estrogens tend to increase serum thyroxine-binding globulin (TBg). In a patient with a nonfunctioning thyroid gland who is receiving thyroid replacement therapy, free levothyroxine may be decreased when estrogens are started thus increasing thyroid requirements. However, if the patient's thyroid gland has sufficient function, the decreased free thyroxine will result in a compensatory increase in thyroxine output by the thyroid. Therefore, patients without a functioning thyroid gland who are on thyroid replacement therapy may need to increase their thyroid dose if estrogens or estrogen-containing oral contraceptives are given.

Drug/Laboratory Test Interactions: The following drugs or moieties are known to interfere with laboratory tests performed in patients on thyroid hormone therapy: androgens, corticosteroids, estrogens, oral contraceptives containing estrogens, iodine-containing preparations, and the numerous preparations containing salicylates.

Fasting increases absorption. Malabsorption syndromes, as well as dietary factors (children's soybean formula, concomitant use of anionic exchange resins such as cholestyramine), cause excessive fecal loss. T3 is almost totally absorbed, (95% in 4 hours). The hormones contained in the natural preparations are absorbed in a manner similar to the synthetic hormones.

More than 99% of circulating hormones are bound to serum

proteins, including thyroid-binding globulin (TB g), thyroid-binding prealbumin (TBPA), and albumin (TB a), whose capacities and affinities vary for the hormones. The higher affinity of levothyroxine (T4) for both TB g and TBPA as compared to triiodothyronine (T3) partially explains the higher serum levels and longer half-life of the former hormone. Both protein-bound hormones exist in reverse equilibrium with minute amounts of free hormone, the latter accounting for the metabolic activity.

Deiodination of levothyroxine (T4) occurs at a number of sites, including liver, kidney, and other tissues. The conjugated hormone, in the form of glucuronide or sulfate, is found in the bile and gut where it may complete an enterohepatic circulation. Eighty-five percent of levothyroxine (T4) metabolized daily is deiodinated.

## NODULES AND SWELLINGS

Thyroid nodules are swellings or lumps in the gland, which do not usually interfere with the normal activity of the gland. The symptoms are due to the lump itself, which may cause discomfort, or press on the gullet behind, causing swallowing difficulties. Very rarely a lump may also press on the windpipe causing breathing difficulties. Most patients however only notice the lump incidentally; it can be too small to cause symptoms.

**There are however several types of nodule.**

1.   *Thyroid Cyst.*
*This is just a fluid filled swelling, which is of no*

*significance. It can be drained by sticking a needle into it and withdrawing the fluid. Monitor with underarm and pulse testing.*

### 2. <u>Multiple Cysts (Colloid)</u>
*This is a collection of many small cysts, and is of no importance. If very large the NHS usually offer surgery. Again try changing your lifestyle and thyroid supplements.*

### 3. <u>Hot Nodule</u>
*This is a small part of the thyroid gland which is working independently from the rest of the gland. If it is producing excess thyroid hormone it is known as a 'hot nodule' and this may cause 'hyperthyroidism'. It needs to be treated like other causes of hyperthyroidism by supporting both the thyroid and adrenals and changing diet.*

### 4. <u>Thyroid Adenoma</u>
*This is a benign growth. Surgical removal is usually advised because there is a small risk it could become malignant in the future. First treat with natural thyroid and remove all chemicals from environment.*

### 5. <u>Thyroid Cancer</u>
*There are various forms of carefully under a microscope. If the lump is a cyst, then the fluid can be removed.*

*Some nodules can become thyroid cancers, but the majority of them are slow growing with a relatively good outcome after treatment. Some are readily curable. Treatment would require surgery and often high dose radioactive iodine. I don't know anyone who has had this treatment and is happy.*

## Investigations which may be used to tell the doctor whether the lump needs treated or not

***a)*** **Blood tests** *– these are important to check whether the gland is working normally.*

***b)*** **X-ray and Ultrasound** *– these are painless and provide pictures of the gland, the lump and the tissue around the gland.*

***c)*** **Radioisotope Scan** *– This provides a picture of the thyroid lump but also gives an indication whether the lump is making lots of thyroid hormone ('hot nodule') or none at all ('cold nodule').*

**d)** **Fine needle aspiration** – this is usually the most helpful investigation. The needle which is used is the same size as that used for blood tests (i.e. quite small!) and is passed into the lump. If the lump is solid then cells from the lump are removed, and examined carefully under a microscope. If the lump is not solid then it should respond easily to treatment, but may take a few months to completely heal.

**Note: thyroid supplements should be used before any surgery. Usually the lumps go when on the correct dose.**

Thyroid nodules are growths of cells in the thyroid gland. These growths can be noncancerous (benign) or cancerous (malignant). Some nodules are fluid-filled (cysts), while others are made of thyroid gland cells. Sometimes, what feels like one nodule will actually be a collection of small nodules.

Thyroid nodules are more common in women than in men. A person's chance of a thyroid nodule increases as we age and the thyroid function decreases. Only a few thyroid nodules are cancerous.

The following characteristics increase the chances that a thyroid nodule is cancerous:  A hard nodule. A nodule that is stuck to nearby structures. One of the causes may be a history of thyroid cancer through various (not all) generations.

You may at first notice a change in your voice it may be hoarse due to vocal cord paralysis. It can affect any age, but over 70's may be at a higher risk. A history of radiation exposure to the head or neck can also be a cause, if affects both sexes.

Causes of thyroid nodules are not always found, but can include: Hair dye, chemicals onto the head, poor protein diet. Hashimoto's disease; or iodine deficiency in your diet.

Do not go down the surgery route before trying thyroid supplements. You will need to take them after surgery regardless.

# THYROID WEIGHT TABLE GUIDE

There is a much simpler way to get thyroid supplementation right for the individual and that's weight. If you weigh:

7 stones the dose is usually 75mcgs of T4,
8 stones 100mcgs,
9 stones 125mcgs,
10 stones = 150mcgs,
11 = 175mcgs,
12 = 200mcgs,
13stones = 225mcgs,
14 stones = 250mcgs,
15 stones = 275mcgs,
16 stones = 300mcgs and so on.

The starting dose, frequency of dose titration, and the optimal full replacement dose should be based on several key parameters including:
(1) Patient age - e.g. older patients: start lower and monitor daily for 3 months
(2) Weight (1.6-1.7 mcg/kg lean body weight). Note: based on available research
(3) Cardiovascular status (positive history of coronary artery disease warrants initiation at a very low dose and very slow titration),
(4) General health.
(5) Concomitant medications (see examples below).
(6) Severity and duration of hypothyroidism.

Consultation with an endocrinologist should be considered in the following cases:
(1) Patients less than 18 years old. (2) Patients

unresponsive to therapy.  (3) Pregnant patients.  (4) Cardiac patients.  (5) Presence of goiter, nodule, or other structural changes in the thyroid gland.  (6) Presence of other endocrine disease.  (7) Patient's receiving amiodarone or other complicating concomitant therapy (8) Stupor, coma.

Because lean body weight (LBW) - [Total body weight minus the weight of all body fat] is difficult to estimate, ideal body weight (IBW) frequently has been used....

Estimated ideal body weight in (kg)
Males: IBW = 50 kg + 2.3 kg for each inch over 5 feet.
Females: IBW = 45.5 kg + 2.3 kg for each inch over 5 feet

**The goal of replacement therapy is to achieve and maintain a clinical and biochemical euthyroid state**. The goal of suppressive therapy is to inhibit growth and/or function of abnormal thyroid tissue. The dose of Synthroid/Thyroxine that is adequate to achieve these goals depends on a variety of factors including the patient's age, body weight, cardiovascular status, concomitant medical conditions, including pregnancy, concomitant medications, and the specific nature of the condition being treated.
(See package insert information for WARNINGS and PRECAUTIONS). Hence, the following recommendations serve only as dosing guidelines.

**Dosing must be individualized and adjustments made based on periodic assessment of the patient's clinical response and laboratory parameters.**

Synthroid/Thyroxine is administered as a single daily dose, preferably one-half to one-hour before breakfast. Synthroid/Thyroxine should be taken at least 4 hours apart from drugs that are known to interfere with its absorption. Due to the long half-life of levothyroxine, the peak therapeutic effect at a given dose of levothyroxine sodium may not be attained for 4-6 weeks. Caution should be exercised when administering Synthroid/Thyroxine to patients with underlying cardiovascular disease, to the elderly, and to those with concomitant adrenal insufficiency.

TSH goal is 1 – 2 on the range chart; however 0.03 is common when the patient is on the correct dose.

## IMPROVE YOUR BRAIN FUNCTION AND IMPROVE YOUR MOOD

**Pantothenic acid or vitamin B5** is not only vital for healthy brain function but also adrenal function. It is a stamina enhancer and essential for making steroid hormones, especially cortisol and cortisone. This is particularly important while you are under stress.

**Arginine Pyroglutamate:** A study over a 60 day period sowed significant improvements in memory function. In Italy it is used for mental retardation, senility, and alcoholism. A must for good memory.

**Niacin, vitamin B3** has also been shown to enhance memory functions and thyroid metabolism. Take care to have the non-flushing one, but the flushing does not last for long. It is a direct response to adrenal metabolism.

| DOSES: | LEVEL 1 | LEVEL 2 | LEVEL 3 (maximum) |
|---|---|---|---|
| DMAE | 150MG | 500MG | 1,000MG |
| PANTOTHENIC ACID | 100MG | " | " |
| B3 | 50MG | 150MG | 250MG |
| L-ARGININE pyroglutamate | 150MG | 500MG | 1,000MG |

(I find L-Arginine, a circulation and heart stimulant, too strong at 500mg) If you get tightness or heart irregularities do stop or lower the dose.

## EMOTIONAL HEALTH

It takes a while for the body to re-balance. Think about how long you have felt unwell, and this is usually how long it will take you to feel better. Patience and determination is needed.

Foods are half of the healing it is important to give up the grains, especially wheat. Try and live a healthier lifestyle without the junk food, eat fresh whenever you can. Always be allergy tested first.

Emotions are next, which include stressors. You need to address these as part of your healing it can be work, partner, family, location etc.

Each emotion or feeling has a vibration these affect your wellness.

Emotions are linked to an organ.  In Chinese medicine
the seven primary emotions are:

**Anger**    Rage, Resentment, Frustration = Liver

**Fear**  = Kidneys

**Fright**  = Gallbladder

**Grief**  Sadness = Lung

**Joy**  Over-excitement, Manic

**Worry and Pensiveness**  = Spleen, which in turn affects the heart

You can be broken hearted.

HEALTHY

|     | Joy/Appreciation/Empowered/Freedom/Love |
| --- | --- |
| 1.  |                                         |
| 2.  | Passion                                 |
| 3.  | Enthusiasm/Eagerness/Happiness          |
| 4.  | Positive Expectation/Belief             |
| 5.  | Optimism                                |
| 6.  | Hopefulness                             |
| 7.  | Contentment                             |

*MODERATE*

|     |                                     |
| --- | ----------------------------------- |
| 8.  | *Boredom*                           |
| 9.  | *Pessimism*                         |
| 10. | *Frustration/Irritation/Impatience* |
| 11. | *Overwhelment*                      |
| 12. | *Disappointment*                    |
| 13. | *Doubt*                             |
| 14. | *Worry*                             |
| 15. | *Blame*                             |
| 16. | *Discouragement*                    |

POOR

|     |                                             |
| --- | ------------------------------------------- |
| 17. | Anger                                       |
| 18. | Revenge                                     |
| 19. | Hatred/Rage                                 |
| 20. | Jealousy                                    |
| 21. | Insecurity/Guilt/Unworthiness               |
| 22. | Fear/Grief/Depression/Despair/Powerlessness |

| Human Emotion | | Energy Frequency |
|---|---|---|
| 40.0 | Serenity of Being | Ultra-high |
| 30.0 | Postulates | Frequency |
| 20.0 | Action | |
| 8.0 | Exhilaration | |
| 6.0 | Aesthetic | Very-high |
| 4.0 | Enthusiasm | Frequency |
| 3.5 | Cheerfulness | |
| 3.3 | Strong Interest | |
| 3.0 | Conservatism | |
| 2.9 | Mild Interest | High |
| 2.8 | Contented | Frequency |
| 2.5 | Boredom | |
| 2.4 | Monotony | Low |
| 2.0 | Antagonism | Frequency |
| 1.9 | Hostility | |
| 1.8 | Pain | |
| 1.5 | Anger | |
| 1.4 | Hate | |
| 1.3 | Resentment | |
| 1.2 | No Sympathy | |
| 1.15 | Unexpressed Resentment | |
| 1.1 | Covert Hostility | |
| 1.05 | Anxiety | |
| 1.0 | Fear | Very-low |
| 0.98 | Despair | Frequency |
| 0.96 | Terror | |
| 0.9 | Sympathy | |
| 0.8 | Propitiation | |
| 0.5 | Grief | |
| 0.4 | Making Amends | |

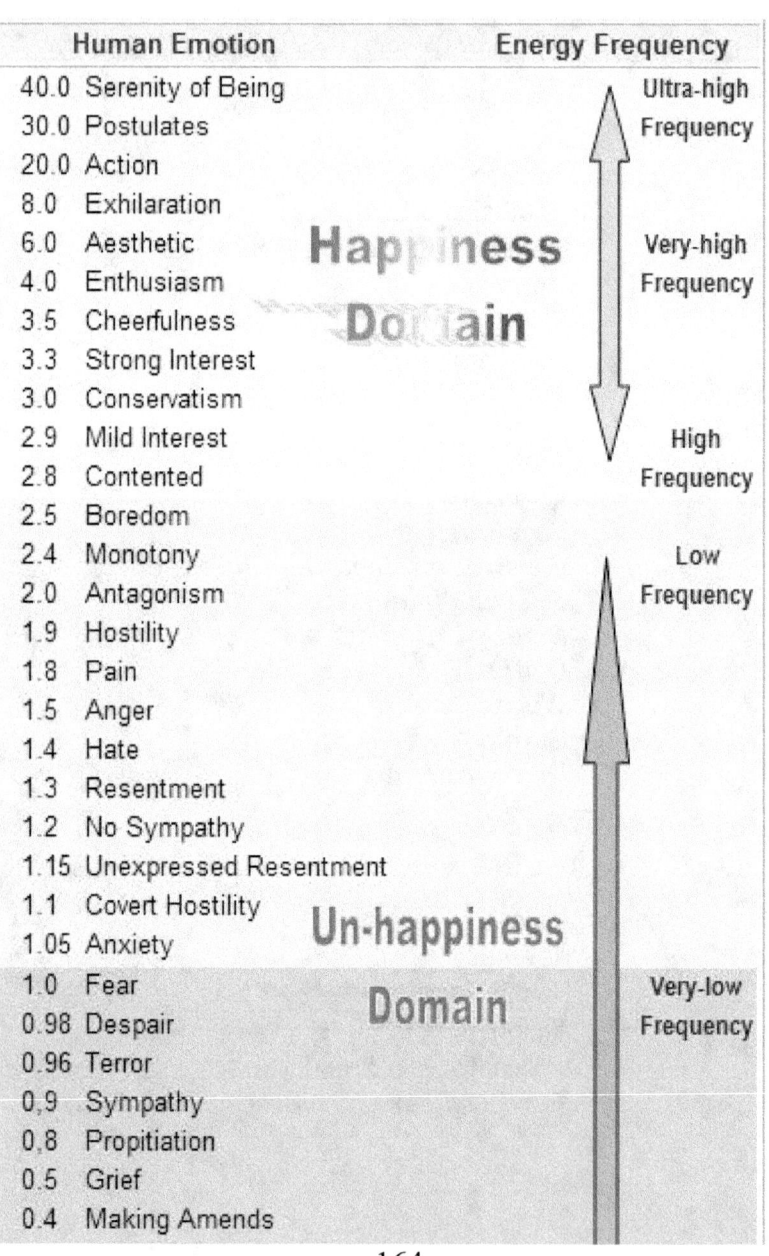

Happiness Domain

Un-happiness Domain

# INFORMATION SHEETS

## LIST OF SIGNS AND SYMPTOMS

**PHYSICAL:**

**Exhaustion:** falling asleep - wanting to go to sleep all the time, weight gain.

**Puffiness of:** eyes  face  hands  feet  ankles

**Pain in:**  head  migraines, lower back pain, neck pain, muscle pain and joints aching.

**Cramps:**  pins and needles. Leg pains at night.

**Skin:** dry flaky course patches, sallow in colour, pallor: flushed/ normal, palms and hands red and burning, itchy hands and feet and skin generally

**Nails:**  brittle, flake off, soft slow growing, thick toenails. Ridges

**Ears:** deafness, over-sensitive hearing, noises in ears, whistling in ears, aversion to loud noise.

**Numbness in:**  toes fingers arms legs back of head, (top and back)

**Eyes:** Visual disturbances: blurring poor focusing dry eyes gritty eyes sore eyes itchy eyes  heavy (hooded) eyelids yellow bumps on eyes.

**Digestive problems:** Loss of appetite food sensitivity food allergies wheat intolerance problems with carbohydrate metabolism, alcohol intolerance constipation diarrhea poor food absorption, pain in liver area, gassy tummy, lots of wind

**Hair:** loss thinness, loss of outer third of eyebrows, lank greasy flat to head (no body), loss of under arm hair and pubic hair, no shine - dull falling out.

**Menstrual disorders:** heavy periods painful periods loss of periods, irregular periods infertility light scant periods loss of sex drive,

**Energy:** slow movements, unable to walk far, low energy, slow speech,

**Blood pressure:** high or low or normal dizziness fainting feeling, palpitations light sensitive sun sensitive balance problems Intolerance of heat and cold, prone to overheating and hot flushes, feet cold, unable to get warm even with jumpers on. Insomnia nightmares, unable to sleep deeply and wake refreshed, (this can be liver)

**EMOTIONAL:**

**Mental:** Panic attacks, poor memory especially short term, concentration poor, word confusion noises and voices in the head, hallucinations, claustrophobia phobias fearfulness, don't want to go out. Poor mood and or low self esteem.

**Emotions:** cry easily, mood swings, unable to be rational, angry, think everyone's against you, depressed nervous anxious persecution complex, personality changes resentfulness towards partners/family/friends/others suspicion of others motives, lack of confidence, wanting to be alone

## HOMEOPATHIC MEDICINE INFORMATION SHEET

Thanks to new technology it is now possible to make up a homeopathic remedy to suit the individual. The dilution and frequency varies from blood group and rhesus.

Ideally a total test would be the best way to see what the baseline is. However a mini scan can be done from the person's human hair. The formula to balance that person is made to measure.

Most people will know that homeopathy works by giving the body a minute dose of medicine to stimulate the body to work by itself again – naturally. If you work out how long you have been ill for – or how long it took you to become very ill – you can then work out how long it may take you to heal. Faith and patience is needed. However most people feel better after a couple of weeks and it is common for them to improve after a few days.

167

Many things cause the body to be imbalanced. Emotions and or stress can be the cause. Often foods are the culprit. Most people do not see food as a medicine (i.e. food = feeding the body, soul and spirit). One example of this is those people who have visited clinics who had poor bowel flora, and needed a remedy to clean out parasites.

Pharmaceutical medicine often makes a person worse – you only have to read the contra indications in the NIMS to see that. It is possible to check this for balance using EAV testing. The computer will show if your medicine is balancing, weakening, or strengthening you. It does this by reading through the electrodes your reaction to the medicine. The test requires the person to be as natural as possible for the best results. GSR is used for the stress test by using a wand in one hand - painless.

## A GENERAL GUIDE TO TAKING
## ENERGETIC HOMEOPATHIC MEDICINE

# Please read very carefully

**ENERGETIC MEDICINE is not the same as classical homeopathy**
This unique medicine uses string theory in quantum physics to help you to heal yourself (no one else can do this). The energy between the electrons and protons is called string energy. It is so small it can

only be detected with specialist equipment. You are always aware of the energy, often sensing it. Because it cannot be seen does not mean it does not exist. The energy needed for each person varies, and the dose is made to help you to heal. We are all made differently, and require specially designed energy to help balance us. Our blood groups also have a great impact on which frequency is best. Blood group O balances best on 10C

The energetic homeopathic is made by imprinting the correct frequencies into water. Water has the same composition as blood, making it the best way to convey the energy. Only pure boiled spring water is used.

**Substances which interfere with homeopathic medicine**: nicotine, excess alcohol in any form, coffee, tea, chocolate, sugar, carbonated drinks, mint, other homeopathic remedies, essential oils, decaffeinated items.

Mint in particular has a neutralizing effect; this can be toothpaste, chewing gum etc.

Garlic, onions, leeks and other sulphur foods affect its' effectiveness

Strong fumes, such as perfumes, body products, sprays, chemicals, deodorants etc.

ALWAYS TAKE YOUR HOMOEPATHIC UPON WAKING AND KEEP AWAY FROM ALL SYNTHETIC CHEMICALS FOR 20 MINUTES. Take nothing orally for 20 minutes, and that includes toothpaste.

Tap the bottle on your palm a few times to re-energise. DO NOT ALLOW THE STOPPER TO TOUCH YOUR MOUTH. Release the drops under your tongue and hold for a few second before swallowing.

DO NOT TAKE OTHER HOMEOPATHICS WITH YOUR ENERGETIC MEDICINE

Do not open bottles near fumes of any kind, such as perfumes, sprays etc.

ALWAYS STORE THE BOTTLE OUT OF DIRECT SUNLIGHT IN A CUPBOARD. **IT IS VITAL THE BOTTLES ARE NOT STORES NEAR ELECTRICITY OR APPLICANCES.**

When flying do not allow medicine to go through X-ray machines, cover in foil. DO NOT USE OR STORE NEAR MOBILE PHONES.

Homeopathics do not interfere with conventional drugs. They are safe and cannot harm you. The healing is slow and gentle. Please be patient.

## General rules about taking homeopathic medicine:

1. take nothing by mouth 15 mins before taking the dose includes all foods, medicines, toothpaste, drinks, cigarettes chewing gum etc. avoid coffee, caffeine, nicotine, carbonated drinks, chocolate – these are drugs and should be avoided – if you must have these leave for one hour after taking the drops. Take note that they my hinder your healing.
2. no mint in any form – toothpaste, chewing gum, or food.
3. no camphor – rubs or orally
4. avoid fumes of all sorts DIY etc.
5. avoid chemicals
6. keep medicine out of sunlight or fridge
7. **no fluoride**
8. no foil or aluminum
9. NO **Smoking or alcohol** for six weeks – give them up totally
10. no drugs
11. Do not eat industrial food – if it is made in a factory avoid it

**AVOID MARGARINE** PLEASE – butter and natural oils are usually fine. Always be allergy and intolerance tested first any good kinesiologist can do this. For maximum healing eat only fresh foods that you prepare yourself. If any food has more than one ingredient do not buy it.

# BLOOD TESTS – GENERAL INFORMATION

The thyroid gland makes two primary hormones T4 and T3 - it also makes calcitonin, which regulates calcium in the body in conjunction with the parathyroids. More T4 is usually made than T3. T3 is five times more concentrated than T4. The two functions of these hormones are different. T4 has four iodine atoms - like ears - and is responsible for cell regeneration, and temperature control. T3 is converted from T4 in the liver and its primary function is energy. T4 is bound to a thyroid protein initially, which is called TT4 (total T4). Oestrogen is also at times bound to T4 and a TT4 blood test includes this binding. For example women on HRT - oestrogen –may have elevated blood results. This is because under the microscope the thyroid hormone sits on the back of oestrogen and looks like crystal. It is true that the thyroid needs a LITTLE oestrogen to carry it around the body, however too much drowns it and stops it from working because it blocks T4 - T3 conversion in the liver. When the hormones T4 and T3 are unbound to proteins they are free and the blood test for this is FT4 and FT3. Free means that the hormone is available for cell use, and whole body metabolsm.

The pituitary gland within the centre of the brain produces TSH, which is thyroid stimulating hormone. When an outside delivery of T4 is introduced (like Thyroxine), TSH reduces to below

0.0 level e.g. your TSH result if you take Thyroxine may be 0.03. The range is 0.5 - 6.0, the average being 2.9. This test is commonly done by biochemists in the lab. as a prime indicator of PRIMARY hypothyroidism - i.e. when the thyroid is out of control the TSH is high because the pituitary gland is trying to stimulate the thyroid into action. Biochemists are now saying that is TSH is within the range there is no need to do any further testing and that your thyroid is working all right.

A quote from Medicine International reads; "The TSH levels are normal in approximately 50% of patients with secondary hypothyroidism but TT4 and FT4 are usually low".

Another quote on TSH this time from the Department of Health, London reads "If there is a change greater than 0.8 that is significant". The problem with this statement is that most of us do not have a baseline test when we are well, so no one knows what the rise or fall is.

Reference ranges are supplied to give guidance to our doctors and have been designed by a 95% population sample in the 1950's when blood tests were first introduced. One problem with this is that thanks to oil we now live in an oestrogen dominated world, where our food is packaged in plastic, we burn oil as fuel and live in a highly polluted world. Oestrogen dominance stops the thyroid from working properly.

173

The second blood test that should be done is the
FT4 one. The range is 10 - 24. The average is 17.
A double blind trial at Birmingham University in
1997 concluded the following:
1) Those with hypothyroid symptoms fell in the 10
- 14 range
2) Those diagnosed with M.E. fell into the 14 - 16
range
3) Those normal fell into the 17 - 24 range.

TT4 is often done by outdated labs. Many common
medicines affect this test and TT4 is futile in many
cases.

Reasons for laboratory testing are:
1] To confirm the clinical diagnosis
2] To monitor patients who have been treated
3] To select removal of the thyroid gland

TSH testing may be affected by steroidal drugs. Or
sometimes by a tumour of the pituitary gland.

The most common diagnosis is one of elevated TSH
in conjunction with low T4.

The thyroid gland also makes thyroid binding
proteins. Asprin destroys this simple action. Free
thyroid levels represent less than 1% of the total
number of thyroid hormones in the bloodstream.

The FT4 test in theory should by total T4 multiplied by T3 resin uptake and should be proportional to free T4.

FT3 is very rarely done. The conversion of T4 to T3 in the liver by growth hormone is largely ignored by the medical profession.

Eighty percent of people who contact the group are diagnosed hypothyroid but still unwell because they are monitored by blood testing. The amount of Thyroxine in the blood stream does not equate to having a level high enough to make you feel well. Indeed some people are toxic to Thyroxine and need Tertroxin T3 for their energy.

The TT4 test range is 50 - 160; your result may be 90. Mine was and I felt terrible. But was it really 90 or was it lower because I was on a high dose of pharmaceutical HRT?

Under the Patients Charter you are entitled to see or have a photocopy of your blood test. If anyone tells you it is normal get a copy and we will interpret it for you.

Some things to NEVER DO before a blood test: take any supplements for 36 hours prior to the test, drink caffeine, alcohol, or have any stimulant. Chocolate can alter it. Make sure that you do not wash your hair because alum in shampoos affects blood tests. Never be tested in the morning because your hormones are at their highest then. Cortisol interacts with thyroid hormones and it declines as the day progresses. You can have a blood test and have another five minutes later and there can be 10 points difference between them.

Finally the report caried out by the Audit Commission in December 1998 states that "50% of laboratories provide false test results. One doctor sent two samples out of the same arm and needle with two different names on to test the lab. They both came back with different results.

Blood tests vary so much they cannot be relied upon. Temperature and pulse with signs and symptoms are a much better way forward with diagnosis.

Your doctor should gently finger-tip examine your thyroid whilst standing behind you. If it is swollen or lumps can be felt then thyroid medication should be recommended. Staring with a low dose and increasing by 1/4 tablet every four days until your pulse and temperature are normal. Readings of 17 on the T4 range are recommended.

## WERE YOU EVER TESTED WHEN YOU WERE "NORMAL"?

# PITUITARY GLAND

The pituitary gland is a small pea sized endocrine gland located in the bone of the brain stem.  The gland is attached to the hypothalamus by a stalk and, if undamaged, there is a negative feedback system operating between the two.  The hypothalamus is located behind the eyes, which is often where we get a headache.

The pituitary/hypothalamus system operates to control our important body functions, such as temperature, appetite, metabolism, water balance, sleeping/waking cycle, periods, sexual activity etc.  The pituitary then co-ordinates everything it is like a master conductor.

Vitamin A affects the pituitary function greatly.  The thyroid is controlled by the pituitary.  It produces TSH - thyroid stimulating hormone.  This TSH rises and falls to accommodate your thyroids needs.  TSH makes sure that the blood has enough thyroid hormones to service the living cells.  When the correct level is reached TSH shuts off via the negative feedback system.  Vitamin A deficiency throws this out of kilter and iodine uptake is reduced along with TSH.  Low Vitamin A can reduce thyroid function of up to 50%.

Secondary hypothyroidism is often caused by either a pituitary malfunction, adrenal insufficiency or severe illness.  A car accident - whiplash - can

177

damage the pituitary itself and the nerves and blood vessels to it.  Or perhaps a tumor could cause a malfunction however this is very rare.

The structure of the pituitary gland is divided into - two the anterior and the posterior.  The posterior is attached to the hypothalamus.  The anterior makes major hormones, which control the endocrine system and bodily functions.  FSH is follicle stimulating hormone, which controls egg development in the ovaries in women and sperm production in men.  LH is lutenising hormone, which controls egg release and testosterone secretion.  Growth hormone controls glucose production and liver function.  TSH control thyroid function.  Prolactin stimulates breast milk.  ACTH sends messages to the adrenal cortex to produce cortisol.

Low Growth Hormone is indicated by obesity, poor and thin skin, low energy levels, osteoporosis, and diabetes.

FSH is blood tested to show if oestrogen levels are too low.  Often they are too high which indicates that the menopause is onset.  Likewise LH is tested for natural progesterone and menopause onset.

The posterior pituitary outputs ADH which is antidiuretic hormone, also called vasopressin.  If thyroid function is working properly then this hormone also works to control fluid function.

Swollen ankles and fingers are an indicator that it is not working properly. Excess salt affects this hormone adversely. Have a sodium test with a thyroid blood test.

Oxytocin controls uterus contractions and plays an important role in lactation. Anyone breast-feeding will recognize the connection between suckling and after pains or the uterus going back to its normal size.

Many women with hypothyroidism are infertile because the pituitary does not control the release of eggs properly. Periods are often out of sinc. The can be heavy or scant because of pituitary malfunction. Treatment with natural thyroid usually re-balances this. The cessation of ovulation causes the pituitary to compensate by sending messages to release large quantities of FSH and LH because the ovaries produce a hormone which balances iodine this is often the point when women begin to feel ill and develop hypothyroidism.

The importance of natural progesterone on the pituitary is ignored. If progesterone is too low then the pituitary compensates by releasing high levels of FSH and LH. This in turn produces more oestrogens and the circle continues. Low progesterone = depression e.g. after child birth. During pregnancy progesterone levels are extremely high but after the birth the drop sharply and many women experience post-natal depression. Some do not recover. Low progesterone levels can lead to hypothyroidism.

Polycystic ovaries are often the cause of poor pituitary function and or poor thyroid function.

How can we keep out pituitary glands working properly? The answer is an almost impossible task. Many people develop secondary hypothyroidism because they have had a shock. Bereavement is high on the list. The stress response becomes exhausted in the adrenals resulting in pituitary malfunction. ACTH cannot keep up with prolonged stress. Meningitis and infection also affects the pituitary - the virus destroying the cells. We could try and keep out of the car. Whiplash throws the head back and the pituitary is banged inside the bone (where it lives), causing irreparable damage. It would help is we could keep out of the operating theatres where anaesetic kills pituitary cells. We could decline from taking the Pill and other pharmaceutical medications, especially steroids, which long term affect both thyroid and pituitary function. And finally we could eat a sensible diet. Avoid taking aspartame in foods and drink, no fizzy drinks and processed foods. Aspartame is in yogurt and so many other industrial foods. Always check you foods for additives. Aim for stevia as a sweetener, which is a natural plant.

Keep your pituitary healthy by avoiding chemicals, especially conditioner on clothes and hair.

# DIET FOR A HEALTHY LIFE

Unless you have food allergies the following diet is recommended: all should be organic where possible. ***YOU SHOULD ALWAYS BE FOOD TESTED FIRST BEFORE EMBARKING ON ANY DIET. Not all foods are good for all people. What balances you will be different to another person because we are individuals and although we share genes we are not clones of each other.***

Apples (if washed + peeled) 1 per day
Apricots
Avocados twice per week
Bananas 2– 3 per week
Blackberries, blackcurrents, elderberries, redcurrents, raspberries, cranberries
Black pepper and sea salt
Brocolli   once a week
Full Milk
Butter   250gr per week
Carrots
Celery
Dandelion,
Dill, rosemary, tarragon, fennel, yam, basil, bay, sage
Ginger - raw root
Gooseberry
Extra virgin olive oil or regular
Fish whenever you feel like it
Free range eggs maximum ten per week

Fresh herbs – soak in sea salt – daily
Freshly squeezed/juiced fruit and vegetable juice
Glucose 1 tsp when energy levels are too low
Grapes if washed thoroughly
Grapeseed oil
Herb teas, thyroid/adrenals support tea, ginger tea for adrenals
Herbs – damiana, mint
Lemons half per day
Peaches,
Plums
Lettuce, flat hothouse organic
Live - bio yogurt at night
Liver once per week
Pears - best cooked
Maduki Honey
Mango
Meat, game and poultry daily
Minerals - selenium, zinc, magnesium, iron
Nuts (No Brazils or peanuts) twice per week
Oily fish twice per week
Papaya                    Pineapple
Red wine twice per week (one small glass)
Spinach
Spring water - check mineral water for nitrates, flouride and sulphates, always boil first.
Strawberries                Sweet potatoes
Vegetable oil
Vegetables – not the cabbage family
Vitamins - all the B's C, E, folic acid, D (No multi-vitamins).
Yams

It is easy to follow a simple food protocol.

Have one day off when you eat what you want, know that you may feel ill the following two days

Your plate should be the size of your open hand

Your oils and good fats at each meal should be 1 fluid ounce

Your salt intake should be no more than ¼ teaspoon daily

Your protein at each main meal should cover the palm of our hand

Your vegetables should be the size of your fist

You should drink a glass of good quality water before eating not after

Your food should be cooked from fresh

Avoid all additives and industrial factory prepared food

The rule of thumb is that if food has more than one ingredient avoid it.


See: "A Thyroid and Hormone Diet"- for more details.

# DHEA

Main primary hormone

DHEA is one of the most important hormones in the blood stream, and has been shown to be one of the primary factors in aging and age related diseases. As we age our DHEA levels decrease.

Nearly 5,000 in-depth scientific and medical studies on the use of DHEA have been conducted and completed in the laboratories of some of the top universities and medical research facilities in the world (BioTech News).

DHEA is rapidly becoming known as the anti-aging miracle of the 21st century

DHEA levels are directly related to mortality in humans (Dr Ward Dean, MD, Smart Drug News).

Current research suggests that DHEA may be of value in preventing and treating cardiovascular disease, high cholesterol, diabetes, obesity, cancer, Alzheimer's disease, other memory disturbances, and immune system disorders including chronic fatigue.

DHEA may also enhance the body's immune response to viral and bacterial infections...New evidence suggests this hormone is so beneficial that it may turn out to be the most important medical advance of the decade(Dr Alan R. Gaby, MD).

DHEA is specifically formulated to slow release to assure the benefit of maximum absorption.

# What Is DHEA?

Dehydroepiandrosterone, or DHEA, is a steroid hormone, a chemical cousin of testosterone and estrogen. It is made from cholesterol by the adrenal glands, which sit atop each kidney. For the first few years of life, the adrenals make very little DHEA. Around age six or seven, they begin churning it out. Production peaks in the mid-20s, when DHEA is the most abundant hormone in circulation. From one's early '30s on, there's a steady decline in DHEA production, so the average 75-year-old has only 20% of the DHEA in circulation that he or she had 50 years earlier. At all ages, men tend to have higher DHEA levels than women.

By definition, hormones are chemical messengers made in a gland or tissue that start, stop, or otherwise orchestrate activity in some other issue. That makes DHEA a hormone in name only, since no one knows exactly what it does in the body. For years it was thought to be a kind of chemical trash left over from making other hormones. Today, "we still haven't been able to identify any mechanism of action," says Dr. Casson. In fact, about the only thing that researchers can agree on is that DHEA is easily converted into other hormones, especially estrogen and testosterone.

FDA
Ten years ago the agency told companies to stop selling DHEA, which was marketed at the time for weight loss, and classified it as an unapproved new drug, obtainable only by prescription. Then in 1994, DHEA was reclassified as a dietary supplement, allowing sales over the counter.

# THE EVIDENCE

Much of DHEA's reputation as a wonder hormone comes from experiments in which mice or rats were fed daily doses. Such studies have shown that DHEA can prevent or delay the onset of cancer, "hardening" of the arteries, lethal viral infections, lowered immunity, obesity, and diabetes. But what works in rodents doesn't necessarily work in humans. That may be especially true in this case, because rats and mice produce only about 1/10,000 the DHEA we do. An early human study that pointed to possible benefits for DHEA came from Dr. Barrett-Connor's group. They measured DHEA levels in blood samples taken from almost 2,000 men and women between 1972 and 1974 and looked at how many died from heart disease. In 1986, they reported that men with high DHEA levels were far less likely to have died of heart disease, while women with high DHEA levels were at greater risk. A more detailed analysis published late last year, however, showed that men with above-average DHEA levels back in the early 1970s were only 15% less likely to have died of heart disease, while there was no association between DHEA levels and heart disease in women. The longest and perhaps most carefully conducted work in humans comes from Dr. Yen and his associates. In their latest study, published last year in a special issue of the Annals of the New York Academy of Sciences devoted to DHEA and aging, eight men and eight women aged 50 to 65 took either 100 milligrams of DHEA or an identical placebo pill each night for three months. For three months after that, they took the opposite pill. Within two weeks of starting DHEA, circulating levels of the hormone were a bit higher than normally found in young adults. Lean body mass increased slightly in both sexes, as did muscle strength, which also improved with the placebo. Fat body mass decreased in men but increased a bit in women.

There was also a rise in some chemical markers that suggested improvement in immune function, though the number of colds and other illnesses was not measured.

An earlier study from Dr. Yen's group showed that three months of daily 50-milligram doses of DHEA significantly improved the sense of "well-being," it did not improve sex drive, as advertisements for DHEA often claim.

Another study in which volunteers took DHEA suggests that this hormone may help treat the autoimmune disease lupus. Trials looking at DHEA's ability to boost the immune system and maintain mental function in older adults are in progress. Experiments on a few dozen people over six months hardly constitute proof that a treatment works. "What we really need at this point are some long-term clinical trials to identify clear benefits and risks," says Dr. Nestler.

One reason why such trials are crucial is that DHEA has side effects, some of which may be irreversible. Since DHEA is converted into testosterone, some women who take it grow body or facial hair and, if they are under age 50 or so, can stop menstruating. DHEA has also been shown to decrease levels of HDL ("good") cholesterol in women, and could increase the risk of heart disease, the leading killer of older women. "We have no idea what DHEA might do to the risk of breast cancer," says Dr. Nestler.

In men, the increased levels of testosterone seen with daily DHEA pills could stimulate the growth of a tiny prostate tumor that would otherwise have remained dormant. Excess testosterone could also cause the prostate to enlarge, making urination difficult.

## THE BOTTOM LINE

Much of the popular and scientific interest in DHEA stems from our culture's emphasis on youth. If levels of this hormone decline with age, the thinking goes, we could avoid the health problems that accompany aging -- or even extend our lifespan -- by keeping DHEA levels high. Many people are already taking DHEA just in case this turns out to be true. That wouldn't be a problem if this substance were as safe as vitamin C. But as a potent steroid hormone, DHEA has the potential for far-reaching side effects throughout the body. The rush to take DHEA is a curious paradox, especially when compared with the slow, almost grudging acceptance of hormone replacement therapy for older women. After menopause, hormone supplements that boost dwindling levels of estrogen help prevent osteoporosis and may protect against heart disease. There are also some known or suspected risks with estrogen replacement, such as a possible increase in the risk of breast cancer. Despite mounting evidence that the benefits substantially outweigh the risks, most women in the US choose not to start hormone replacement therapy.

DHEA 1 x 50mgs should ONLY be taken in the afternoon. It keeps you awake so NEVER take after tea time.

It is the energy hormone and is on the banned list for the Olympic athletes.

> IT IS BETTER TO DO THE UNDER ARM TEMPERATURE UPON WAKING TEST SO THAT THE TISSUES CAN BE CHECKED.
>
> PUT A THERMOMETER UNDER YOUR ARMPIT FOR TEN MINUTES UPON WAKING WHEN YOU ARE NICE AND WARM

IMPORTANT   PLEASE READ THIS CAREFULLY

## **NATURAL THYROID COMMENCEMENT THERAPY**

These are general guidelines for taking thyroid replacement therapy:

Remember it entirely replaces your own thyroid production - it does this by reducing TSH (thyroid stimulating hormone) to around 0.03, inducing a welfare state.  All thyroid replacement does this, and it is NOT in addition to your own bodies supply.

The dose and medicine is individual to each person, what suits one will not suit another.  You MUST be tested for the correct dose. **Increase by ¼ tablet daily** until you are at your prescribed level. (You may feel tired until you get to your full dose).  Headaches can also be common for a few days while your pituitary adjusts.

The time for taking medicine varies from person to person. You must try and see what feels best for you.  Traditionally T4 is taken in the morning, however glandular (food state) thyroid also contains T3.  T3 has a body life of 8 hours so it may be wise to **split your dose.**

T4 (thyroid iodine four) has a body life of four days, this means that it takes four days to get into the cells and four days to get out, it may be slightly on either side of four days depending on your energy output.

Do NOT take two days medicine together if you have forgotten a day, just carry on as normal.

You should **monitor yourself each day** by taking your pulse at your wrist with two fingers and not your thumb, if you cannot find your pulse here follow the line down from your ear until you feel it there. The average pottering about pulse is 80 beats per minute. You temperature should be 98.4F or 37C upon waking. Do the under arm temperature test by placing a glass thermometer (shaken down at night) under your armpit prior to rising in the morning for 10 minutes, (yes it does take that long). Remember to write these down, at first you may wish to do these two tests three times a day for a week.

- **WARNING** IF YOUR PULSE GOES OVER 90 BEATS PER MINUTE WHILE RESTING CUT DOWN YOUR THYROID DOSE.

These are overdosing symptoms: palpitations, anginal pain, (over the heart), headaches (you may get these at first), agitation, and excitability. These decline when talking the correct dose.

Do not expect to be well overnight, taking thyroid is not like taking an Asprin, (which you must NEVER do as it stops the binding of the thyroid to carrier protein), the healing is a long slow process; remember how long it took you to become ill. Six months to come out of this illness is normal. Your liver may take up to two years to heal.

You will find that keeping a journal of your sign and symptoms will help you see your recovery process. You may feel tired while increasing your dose, or have a headache. These will pass.

T3 – Cytomel/Tertroxin/Cynomel is different because it is five times stronger and is the energy hormone, please remember it works in 20 minutes and takes eight hours to leave the body, the effects last longer.

### Whole Raw Thyroid Tissue Concentrate from Desiccated Thyroid Glandular - 90 Tablets

Desiccated Thyroid Glandular
Raw Thyroid Tissue Concentrate
140 mg.
AND EXTRA STRONG 200mg - 90 Tablets

Most people balance best on either 5 – 6 regular or 3 – 4 extra strong thyroid tablets daily.

Natural thyroid is concentrated whole raw desiccated thyroid glandular is the genuine therapeutic health supplement that everyone is searching for. It is of such high quality that many professionals recommend our product and even use it themselves with great success.

Please don't make the mistake of confusing thyroid products with the many non-effective or imitation combination products that are on the market.

Natural thyroid contains the whole balanced thyroid spectrum just as it comes from the gland. It is produced in Argentina and New Zealand, using stringent quality control and safety measures. It is derived from free range cattle.

191

Natural thyroid DOES NOT require a prescription because we maintain its valued designation as a dietary supplement. To prevent our product from being classified as a drug under Section 201(g) of the Federal Food, Drug and Cosmetic Act, we are required to inform you that there is no intention, implied or otherwise that represents or infers that our product be used in the cure, mitigation, treatment, or prevention of any disease. We are unable to discuss treatment of medical conditions or compare our product to pharmaceutical drugs.

You have the right to research information and make determinations for yourself. Only you can heal you. Natural thyroid cannot heal you, but it may elevate some of your signs and symptoms. It is not a cure.

Bovine Adrenal glandular is also available. This can balance the adrenals and thyroid. The ratio varies but up to 5 adrenal glandular split into two doses daily can make all the difference.

Recommended regular thyroid use: 5-6 tablets daily (140mg) or as otherwise directed by physician or qualified health care practitioner. Always check the correct dose and suitability using hair analysis. Not all products suit all people and the dose varies. You should monitor yourself using pulse and temperature daily, (80 - 84 BPM and 98.4 or 37C).

Each tablet supplies:
Raw Thyroid Concentrate: Other Ingredients: Dicalcium Phosphate, Magnesium Stearate (tablet binders),

Pharmaceutical Glaze: Contains no sugar, starch, salt, wheat, corn, yeast, or soy derivatives.

Tissue processed by Low Temperature Method, to insure rawness and preserve natural constituents.

Natural thyroid is best stored in a cool place for wholesale amounts you can freeze. DO NOT RE-FREEZE.

## WARNING

These statements have not been evaluated by the US Food and Drug Administration (FDA). These products are not intended to diagnose, treat, cure, or prevent any disease.

## ORDERING MEDICINES FROM OVERSEAS

It is possible to order your medicines direct from overseas at lower costs than by private means. An example of this is natural thyroid products. These products retail here at over £60; it is possible to buy them abroad at half the cost.

You are advised to be diagnosed, and have a full knowledge of both the products and your illness. It is known that many people self dose to make themselves feel well enough to function daily - however we advocate that you take only medicines under the control of your doctor or health professional.

### **Disclosure: No liability can be taken for you importing medicines for self use.**

Most Britons on holiday abroad, and discover that they can purchase medicines over the counter from local pharmacies. Thyroxine for example is about £2.00 for 30 in Spain, however take care it does not contain wheat and is Levathroid - remember to ask the pharmacist - most speak English. Remember only 6 in 100 test balanced on this medication alone, most feel unwell when taking it and some are toxic to it. Most people respond best to NTB.

**HOW TO ORDER**

[1]   Remember to <u>only order three months supply</u>. This is a <u>legal requirement</u>. It is also the law that you can only order medicines for **YOURSELF.** There are stringent laws for supplying medicines to others.

[2]   **Keep the price <u>to under £20</u>.** That way you will avoid paying customs, post office handling, and VAT charges. Ask that the customs label be clear about the price and if they are food supplements to state that.

You are strongly advised to be tested first before embarking on the GUESS IT route. This only leads to problems and healing takes much longer.

TAKING THYROID CAN MAKE YOU WORSE for a short period of time. IT IS IMPORTANT TO LEARN ABOUT THE ILLNESS AND WHAT CAUSES IT FIRST. THROWING SOME TABLETS DOWN YOUR THROAT IN THE HOPE THAT YOU MIGHT FEEL BETTER IS STRONGLY NOT ADVISED. You must follow the correct protocol while increasing slowly. Always be tested by a health practitioner first.

Healing should come from all sources, such as food, detoxifications, removal of chemicals from the daily routine. Changes to lifestyle. Emotional healing and exercise.

ALL HEALING SHOULD BE HOLISTIC (whole). Taking tablets for illness drives it further and the body adapts to these in around six months.

You are advised to discover the cause of your illness and not treat the signs and symptoms. Use the hair analysis form. It is an easy way to discover what may be stressing your hormones and how you can help change that.

Always remember these products are dried meat and are food state, no claims are made that they can cure you - however they may help elevate some of your signs and symptoms. Always be checked for suitability, you may be toxic to any of these products and they may make you worse.

## PREGNENOLONE-25 SLOW RELEASE FROM PLANTS

### PREGNENOLONE

**The dynamic Anti-Aging Supplement**
An exciting break though in anti-aging, Pregnenolone a hormone produced by the adrenal glands from cholesterol that is the direct precursor to DHEA. As the bodies own building block of DHEA, Pregnenolone may enhance DHEA's activity and they can be taken together. Pregnenolone is converted directly to Progesterone and so is often an excellent choice for oestrogen-sensitive women or testosterone sensitive men.

Research has shown that Pregnenolone produces other substances in the body, which can greatly improve our resistance to stress and adrenal exhaustion. It has also shown

195

dramatic decreases in fatigue and has been shown to significantly help with PMS and in balancing moods and emotions such as depression and anxiety. Studies have shown Pregnenolone to be hundreds of times more powerful than other memory enhancing substances and have a powerful effect on improving transmission of nerve impulses.

Each tablet contains: 25mg or 50mg of 99% Pure Micronized plant based grade Pregnenolone and is addtitive free

Pregnenolone is a natural hormone made from cholesterol in our adrenal glands. Hormones are the chemical messengers that tell our organs and cells what to do. This "Mother Hormone" is the biological precursor to DHEA also known as the hormone balancer. It has the special ability to increase the levels of steroid hormones which are deficient or reduce and levels of excess circulating hormones. Pregnenolone is synthesized inside our mitochondria, (baby cells), and was found to be the basic precursor for the production of ALL the human steroid hormones, including DHEA, Progesterone, oestrogen, Testosterone, Cortisone, Cortisol and Aldosterone.

*Protection from high cortisol/cortisone: Cortisol levels increase with normal aging causing immune impairment, arteriosclerosis, and neuronal injury. Pregnenolone protects against adrenal atrophy (shrinkage) when withdrawing from cortisone therapy. Pregnenolone helps protect against the effects of elevated cortisol including atrophy of the skin, osteoporosis, arthritis and allergies (it acts as an anti-inflammatory).*

Pregnenolone is only recommended for those over age 50, unless adrenal failure is a major concern.

<u>Pregnenolone and Multiple Sclerosis</u>: Administration of either pregnenolone in mice also promoted myelin (membrane that surrounds our brain and nervous system) formation and repair during nerve regeneration. The degeneration of the myelin sheath is the main problem in multiple sclerosis.

<u>Brain and memory Function</u>: Our neurological function is precisely controlled by hormones that synchronise organ and cell function. Some of the most exciting effects of Pregnenolone is its amazing memory-enhancing effects. Pregnenolone has been found to play a vital role in the acquisition of knowledge and the long-term memory. Several studies have shown that Pregnenolone boosted memory and learning ability in subjects. This neuro-steroid improves the transmission of nerve impulses and facilitates communication between brain cells.

<u>Stress and Fatigue</u>: Many studies have indicated that a daily dose of 50mg of pregnenolone reduced fatigue and stress. It produces adrenal steroids that influence our resistance to stress and help recover our adrenal glands from exhaustion. Other studies indicate that people with chronic depression have only half the levels of Pregnenolone they should have.

Pregnenolone does not seem to have any negative side effects. No reports of side effects have been reported even after decades of use. It is also speculated that pregnenolone is highly discriminative as it converts to other hormones only as they are needed by the body. This reduces the risk for side effects which is sometimes experienced with DHEA and other hormone precursors when taken in excess. It stimulates the thyroid.

# SUPPLEMENT GUIDE

A simple way to get thyroid supplementation right for the individual and that's you morning weight.  If you weigh:

## GENERAL DOSES

7 stones the dose is usually 75mcgs of T4, or 45mcg (300mg per tablet of kelp) or 3/1.5 natural thyroid
8 stones 100mcgs, or 4/2
9 stones 125mcgs, or 5/2.5
10 stones = 150mcgs, or 6/3
11 = 175mcgs, or 7/3.5
12 = 200mcgs, or8/4
13stones = 225mcgs, or 9/4.5
14 stones = 250mcgs, or 10/5
15 stones = 275mcgs, or 11/5 5
16 stones = 300mcgs or 12/6 and so on.
(Note 300mg of pure kelp is equivalent to 15mcg of T4, see table below)

Natural thyroid comes in 2 sizes, 140mg, and 200m.  Adrenal glandular is 100g size.  The ratio is 1:1. (Size = per blood serum volume).

Armour is dispensed in grains, which are equivalent to 60mcgs or the equivalent to 25mcgs of Thyroxine/Synthroid

## WARNING many multi vitamins and minerals contain iodine always check your supplements before taking

| SIZE (stones) | THYROXINE/SYNTHROID | NATURAL THYROID | |
| --- | --- | --- | --- |
| | | Size: 140 | 200 |
| 7 | 75mcgs | 3 | 1.5 |
| 8 | 100 | 4 | 2 |
| 9 | 125 | 5 | 2.5 |
| 10 | 150 | 6 | 3 |
| 11 | 175 | 7 | 3.5 |
| 12 | 200 | 8 | 4 |
| 13 | 225 | 9 | 4.5 |
| 14 | 250 | 10 | 5 |
| 15 | 275 | 11 | 5.5 |
| 16 | 300 | 12 | 6 |

KELP

| Size (stones) | 300mg tablets | T4 |
| --- | --- | --- |
| 7 | 5 x 15 mcgs | 75mcgs of iodine |
| 8 | 7 x 15 | 105 |
| 9 | 8 x 15 | 120 |
| 10 | 10 x 15 | 150 |
| 11 | 11 x 15 | 165 |
| 12 | 13 x 15 | 195 |
| 13 | 15 x 15 | 225 |
| 14 | 16 x 15 | 240 |
| 15 | 18 x 15 | 270 |
| 16 | 20 x 15 | 300 |

What to avoid:

**Overdosing.** It is vital that you get the correct daily dose, and stick to it. NEVER add two or more days together. Remember **it takes 4 days to get T4 into the system**. IT IS VITAL YOU MONITOR YOUR DAILY PULSE AND WAKING

TEMPERATURE. If your resting pulse exceeds 90 beats per minute reduce immediately. You can feel when you are toxic. Always start slowly and increase by a ¼ tablet every other day. When your temperature and pulse are normal stop increasing but continue to monitor daily.

Adrenal glandular can greatly stimulate the thyroid and metabolism. DO NOT ADD adrenal support later, you should do the two together to get the dose right for you. The ratio to natural thyroid varies but you can start with 1:1 tablets per day.

Remember grains interfere with thyroid function and can cause adrenals to be affected. The hyper reaction of insulin can cause you to be toxic.

You are aiming for a pottering about pulse of 80-84 beats per minute. A waking under arm temperaure should be 98.4 or 37C. Your weight should be stable for 2 weeks. You should have a free T4 (FT4), blood test. It should be around 17 in a range of 9 – 24. It's very important to never take thyroid medication or supplements for 24 – 36 hours prior to a blood test as it can cause a false positive. TSH tests are pointless if you take iodine and thyroid supplements. The results are usually 0.03 – the hypothalamus does not need to stimulate the thyroid to make hormones as they are being taken.

Work out your combination therapy to achieve around 17 in the range. If you feel ill taking thyroid medication it may be adrenals that are the problem.

WARNING other medications can greatly affect thyroid metabolism, plus many food types do too. Infection can also affect body temperature. Always consult a health practitioner.

## CHECKING ADRENAL SIGNS AND SYMPTOMS

**The adrenal glands are two hat-shaped orange-colored endocrine glands which are located on the top of both kidneys.** The adrenal glands are triangular shaped and measure about one-half inch in height and 3 inches in length. Each gland consists of a **medulla** (the center of the gland) which is surrounded by the **cortex**. The medulla is responsible for producing epinephrine and norepinephrine (adrenaline). The adrenal cortex produces other hormones necessary for fluid and electrolyte (salt) balance in the body such as cortisone and aldosterone. The adrenal cortex also makes sex hormones but this only becomes important if overproduction is present. They keep you alive. If you look at a diagram in Greys Anatomy you will see that all veins and arteries go to the adrenals, which are central to the cardiovascular system. It is vital that you eat and drink to keep these important little glands alive. Signs of decline are:

Hyperthyroidsim
Constant visits to the toilet – diarrhea
Grey hair
Whistling ears
Headaches
Stomach or digestion problems
Poor sleeping
Vision disturbances
Dark circles under the eyes
Thin top lips

Often when the adrenals start to fail the thyroid test results come back at borderline. If you treat the thyroid and not the adrenals you may not feel well. It may take the thyroid a while, even years, to fall below the bottom range caused by low adrenals.

# WEIGHT LOSS PROGRAMME SIMPLIFIED

Walk everyday for at least 30 minutes 15 minutes out and 15 back, in a green or fresh air place, especially before 10:00 am. A lack of sunlight is implicated in MS. We need one hour of sunlight on our skins daily for vitamin D. This should also increase bone density. Walking stimulates our adrenal glands; the reflexology point for these is on the ball of the foot. The reflexology point for the thyroid is behind the big toe.

Going to bed before 10:00 pm lowers cortisol the stress hormone, also, in deep sleep is where HGH, human growth hormone, is released. HGH regulates our body mass. That is why you should feel so refreshed and in good shape after a good night sleep (among other reasons, of course). Wheat reduces cortisol, causing sleeping problems. Walking for 10 minutes before bedtime helps sleeping. Yoga breathing exercises help.

8 glasses of boiled/cooled spring water per day, (fluoride free and low in nitrates) a cup an hour. Optional add fresh lemon juice for cleansing. Bicarbonate of soda or calcium will alkalize the stomach. Cider vinegar is good for acid problems and candida. Candida and parasites are common in low thyroid. The thyroid regulates the digestion system. Cascara also helps with candida, take 2 at night for a month after doing a parasite cleanse.

No refined carbohydrates, low complex carbohydrates only from vegetables and fruits. Limit/exclude grains, no gluten it inhibits absorption of nutrients by coating the digestive system with glue. 100 grams of good quality protein per day, grains contain less than 8% protein, which interferes with the thyroid protein.

At least 3 fluid ounces of high quality fats and oils 1 fluid ounce x 3 time per day. Essential fatty acids are called this because we die and age without them. For fish oi, it should be natural from the fish itself - be sure it is heavy metal and hexane free. Protein and fat equal new healthy cells. Fats and oils help with the body's communications on all levels and everything is improved by increasing them.

5 – 6 cups of a variety of fresh vegetables each day, not white potatoes. Eat five different brands of vegetables and or fruit per day.

Some form of gentle weight lifting with just 5 lbs is good enough. You just need to be regular with it - at least 3 times per week x 20 minutes.

You should aim at a gradual weight loss or gain, and it can happen by increasing the good things, and decreasing the not so good gradually. The first week your loss should be around half a stone then 2 – 3 lbs each week thereafter. Muscle weighs heavier than fat. Measure 10 points of your body once a week. Weigh yourself in the morning, naked once a week.

Affirmations work incredibly well - for instance, "Everyday in every way I feel better and better." Be happy, say "I feel happy and slim" regularly – out loud.

Stand up tall. Posture is vital, do not slouch. Use yoga stretching for a perfectly toned body.

Do a complete detox before you start your diet, this should be: a] parasite cleanse, 2] kidney cleanse, 3] liver cleanse, 1 week gap then repeat. You can have 2 – 3 stones of parasites living in you. This may make you tired at first.

Obey the rules of the stomach. Always be allergy food, mineral, hormone, and nutrition tested.

A body that is slightly alkaline cannot get ill, Avoid acid foods like grains and nightshade. Do not eat white coloured foods.

Before beginning any diet always be intolerance tested for foods first. Eat breakfast and 3 good meals per day. Snack on fruit/nuts.

Avoid toxic items like caffeine, alcohol, smoking, processed foods and drinks.

Cook only at moderate temperature. Micro-waving kills 70 – 80% of enzymes. Do not use aluminium either for cooking or foil. Keep metals to a minimum. Cook in filtered spring water or rain-water.

Do not buy processed/industrial food. Cook it yourself from local fresh produce.

What you give out you get back, being negative gets negative. Reap and sow good thoughts and emotions. We are what we eat and how we feel. The things that make us ill are trauma, pollution, and parasites.

Use an EMF screener and keep electricity away from you while sleeping. Your bedroom should be a sanctuary.

Keep chemicals away from you and your environment. Use only natural products and clothing.

What fills your life expands. If that is food then you will eat and want more. If you wouldn't do or give it a 3 year old then do not do it or give it to you. Be kind to yourself. Once a week eat and drink what you want.

## Simple to do exercise regime

## <u>QUICK EXERCISES</u>

I recommend you do these either in the **bath**, take care to not have it more than half full. In a warm **bed**; (not before sleeping as they may keep you awake). In a comfortable **chair** preferably in a warm room:

1.  Move 2 inches or 5cm each time
2.  Start with 10
3.  Do not over exercise
4.  Stop if there is any pain
5.  Make sure you are warm before starting
6.  Slowly build up from 10 by 5 or 10 each day to 100
7.  Have one day off

   Start with your feet and work each muscle group upwards. You are lying on your back at first.
   (For all - move them fast for 10 counts and build up each day to 100).

## FEET AND LEGS

1. Place feet in a running up and down position (For all: either on the floor, in the bath or on the bed or chair)
2. Open and close legs, usually a bath width is fine
3. Squeeze buttocks
4. Lift buttocks
5. Lift each leg to chest alternatively, (this gets easier as the week goes on)
6. Move legs and hips back and forward
   (Build up to 500 exercises in total – do them quick, they should take around 8 minutes for this section)

## BUTTOCKS AND LOWER BACK

1. Move hips from side to side
2. Sit up and move hips back and forward
3. Sit up, roll forward and pulse while holding toes with heels up, you can also alternate to pointing the toes
4. Squeeze buttocks and pulse
5. Lift bottom off the floor
   (Build up to 500 exercises in total – do them quick, they should take around 8 minutes for this section)

## STOMACH

1. Sit up, hold elbows and rock back and forward, eventually you will increase the movement to 2 feet back and forward
2. Alternate hands to knees

3. Inhale and hold stomach in count to 10 quick and release
4. Ankles and knees together, inhale and lift buttocks, squeeze and release
(Build up to 500 exercises in total – do them quick, they should take around 5 minutes for this section)

CHEST
1. Put hands together at a right angle to chest and pulse
2. Do scissors with arms
3. Chin stretch, lift head forward a little, knees bent
(Build up to 500 exercises in total – do them quick, they should take around 3 minutes for this section)

ARMS WRISTS AND FINGERS
1. Arms straight over your head and pulse
2. Arms bent in and out forward to shoulder
3. Wave wrists round to left and right alternatively
4. Fingers in and out, turning hands over
5. If sitting up hold arms out and circle palms down alternatively for 50 then change to palms up
(Build up to 100, this section should take 5 minutes)

FACE TONING AND EXERCISE
1. Grin in and out
2. Say mamma and dadda
3. Say the vowels
(Build up daily this section should take 3 minutes)

Finally stand up and do spine twists – arms swinging to the left and right alternatively.

Cool down with shoulder lifts

Remember to breathe evenly as you exercise. Never strain always be gentle to your own capabilities and build up.

Total maximum time: 30 minutes, (usual quick time 15 minutes)

(Do keep topping up the bath water to keep you warm)

These simple exercises can be done by most people, bed bound, chair bound ill and just too exhausted to do the regular ones.

Never strain or over exercise, always take your time and be gentle. It's a good idea if you are very weak to have a mobile phone handy while you bathe.

Putting your wellness protocol together

Planning is the key to success. It is vital that you take care to use each part step by step.

Morning
1. Make sure your supplements are balanced and correct for you
2. Make a 24 hour table
3. Start with waking time
4. Measure under arm temperature, write it down along with sleeping pattern
5. Take homeopathic
6. Have a bath
7. Do your quick exercise regime, building up daily
8. Take relevent supplements
9. Eat a protein and vegetable breakfast

If possible walk to work, or do some housework

Mid morning
Have a snack from the list and water

Lunchtime
1. If possible go for a short walk
2. Eat lunch from food list

Mid afternoon
Have a snack and water

Teatime
Food from list

Evening
Outside yoga breathing exercises

Go to bed at a reasonable time.

Empty all your life of chemicals that are not natural.
Read up on how chemicals interfere with our
hormones.

Take your time and make lifestyle changes to help
you to heal and feel better.  Take responsibility for
your life, it is all about understanding how to be
well, what makes us ill, and being determined to
correct those areas and remove bad habits.

If you do not apply youself to making changes that
are for your own good, then your success will
probably be as limited as the applications you make
to your health.

# AUTHOR'S FINAL NOTE

I have written the book with the sole intention of teaching the reader how to help themselves to become well again. The issues are complex. Our lifestyles and life experiences are so different too. By examining your lifestyle and experiences and learning about the illness I do hope I have helped you to have more knowledge and understanding.

For those who suffer with being overweight try The Hay diet without the carbohydrates. E.g. breakfast would be fruit, bio yogurt, nuts, fruit juice, and herb tea. Lunch – protein, fish or meat or eggs with salad, apples, orange. Dinner should be a mixture of those two.

Some of you will not be overweight hypothyroids but under weight. If you are unable to gain weight stick to the diet, balance your hormones and add Emertia a phyto-oestrogen cream. Some hypothyroids are too thin and this corrects itself once on the correct therapy.

One if the most important aspects of healing is following a protocol which is designed especially for you as an individual. To have this you need to be food, allergy and lifestyle tested. Your medicines, vitamins and supplements need to be checked to see if they balance, weaken or stress you. The EAV and GSR testing are effective means to do this. I don't know anyone who has not improved after using these – provided they carried out the correct protocol. For those small minority who refused to give up their cigarettes, alcohol, had root canal fillings, caps or veneers, toxic supplements etc. They will struggle to get well. For those who have stuck to a healing protocol I have seen them improve dramatically, weight loss is the biggest success. The biological age reduces as the body becomes less stressed and the person looks younger (and feels it). For example a biological age of 80 was reduced to 30 in six weeks. Try it for yourself and see. (A bio age is the rate our cells are multiplying healthily).

The hair analysis protocol is a designer protocol to help the individual heal themselves. It contains recommendations; usually four pages of what may affect you adversely. What suits one person will not suit another, however there is some common ground, as you can see from the information you have read. A general guide is that we can have a gut full of parasites; there may be moulds from grains, fungus from foods, plus all manner of other nasties making us ill. We may have root canal fillings, or a mouth full of metal causing us untold problems. In short it can be absolutely anything that is making you ill and the question is – "What are you going to do about it?" No doctor can heal you, only you can do that. If you think about it logically you got to where you are all by your own doing, and you need to make the decision on how you are going to fix it.

Each person is different – from what we eat to how we feel. Our tastes and feelings are electric vibrational and individual to us. Blanket food advertising does not take this into account. What food suits one person does not suit another – in fact it can make them quite ill. Parasites breed in our gut. We are often riddled with some of the 200 strains of candida and do not know why they get out of control. The answer is that sugar, yeast and starch helps breed them. Old viruses still remain in our system some weaken us; most stress us.

Teeth with amalgam fillings poison us. Each time we bite the fumes from the mercury go into our systems. Root canal fillings block the energy to our glands and organs, affecting all parts of our body and mind. Food fads are bad for us – e.g. low cholesterol equals low hormone levels. Fat does not make us fat; we have a natural cut off point by the liver when we feel full. Try eating a few plates of double cream and see how many you can eat if you don't believe me. Carbohydrate is the common enemy and is so ageing. Carbohydrate exhausts the adrenals and causes allergic reactions in most people creates breathing problems and manufactured products containing carbohydrate are a big problem for us. Most foods contain some carbohydrate – e.g. milk, cheddar cheese etc. An overload of carbohydrate is exhausting and causes poor sleeping patterns.

Each person needs to know what foods to eat, and what to avoid. Which supplements they may need to take, and which to avoid. Not all vitamins suit all people – they can weaken us if taken when not needed.

The objective of this is to balance you in all aspects of life where possible. The healing follows but takes time. A cell does not become well overnight.

May I wish you all the very best of health. There is absolutely no need for you to feel ill all the time. You can take responsibility for your health, and follow a protocol that is designed for you to heal both your body and your life. By placing your faith in others you are dodging the issues. You really do need to place your faith in **yourself.** Find out what foods you can eat, what stresses, balances and weakens you. Find out what medicine works for you, and if you are reading this then the chances are that you are not feeling well on your current medicine. Be intelligent about the problem. Think about discovery and knowledge as a way of healing. I did and it transformed my life. I went from never seeing morning to living in light. From never eating food I enjoyed to a normal diet. From a brain confused and unhappy to an understanding of what does what for me. I realise that as I get older I will not look like a film star or be a brain surgeon or even have a brain like Einstein. My goal in life is to help those who suffer the way that I did – and if I help only one person to get well again then I am happy. Many people ask a wide range of questions about many things, and I believe that if you are honest then that is all they can ask for. The bottom line is if they want to get well, or better than they are then I can help them to understand how to do this. Not everyone wants that help and I respect this. Not every partner wants their loved one to be well.

***ALWAYS REMEMBER THYROID CANNOT WORK WITHOUT PROPER FOODS FOR YOUR BLOOD TYPE, AND OTHER HORMONES TO BALANCE IT.***

© ANGEL HEALTH

www.ingramcontent.com/pod-product-compliance
Lightning Source LLC
Chambersburg PA
CBHW060249290526
45789CB00001B/257